NOW THAT I AM SAVED… WHAT NEXT?

Go to the Next Level

By

D. Vanessa Smith

ISBN: 1-4033-8541-6 (e-book)
ISBN: 1-4033-8542-4 (Paperback)

This book is printed on acid free paper.

1stBooks - rev. 01/10/03

Go to the Next Level...

To get to the next level, you will need to transcend the box in which you began, in order to experience the growth that must occur for you to go to the next level. You will have to allow the Holy Spirit to teach you about things you never heard of before, believe and execute the thoughts into manifestations of your new reality, to be next level material.

Can you do it?...Lets begin.

Table of Contents:

Acknowledgments

I thank the Spirit of the Living God, for His inspiration in putting God's word together in this format to aid new believers and those who want to refresh their walk with God. I also, thank the following Anointed people of God, all the Doctors and Ministers of the Word that have made God's Word clear to all:

Dr. Creflo A. Dollar Jr.
Taffi L. Dollar
Dr. Leroy Thompson Sr.
Joyce Meyers
Dr. Freddrick K. Price
Rev. Franklin Gosnell
Family Radio Station 94.7FM
Dr. T. D. Jakes
Rev. Motley
Believers Voice of Victory
Dr. Rev. David Jefferson Sr.

I also thank, Christopher Divine, Interwide Solutions for Technical Support. I praise God for their obedience to teach and preach the Gospel of Jesus Christ. To instruct us in the way God's word says that we can choose to live and how to take advantage of all of His blessings. May God bless and continue to increase them as they stay faithful to the Word of God.

When I first got Saved...

God called me into the fold while I studied His word during the separation of my first marriage. A girlfriend came by to visit me at mommy's place. She saw the noise and confusion going on all around me, and asked me to come and stay with her for a while, just to sort out my feelings and look at my options. I desperately needed peace and quiet to be with my thoughts, so, I thought. Therefore, I accepted her offer.

I was a Sunday School teacher, for about eight or nine years, but I did not have a personal relationship with God. I knew Mommy had one, and there were people who were at church that had a relationship with God. I even took the classes to get baptized, although I had not received the understanding of scripture, from the Holy Spirit, at that time. I for the most part, would only read, what I had to read, for Sunday School class. Once, I tried to read it straight through like a book, but that did not work. How many of you know, it takes more than just you reading and complaining to have an understanding of scripture?

I did not know, at the time, that the natural man could not understand the ways of God. I was going to church every Sunday, most of the time, after a party or something worst, and I could not understand why, God could not hear my prayers. I did not know, that the prayers of the **righteous** availed much. And the only prayer that God wants to hear from a **sinner** is the prayer of **repentance.**

I was blaming my husband for all the wrong that he did during our marriage. I did not consider that he told me before we got married that he was a woman beater. He told me that he had absolutely **no respect** for credit. He also, told me all about people that have hidden agendas for things, but I was not listening. I just wanted to get married, **by any means necessary.** Sound familiar?

So, while I was in Pam's house, I read a bible I found in church. I figured if someone left it, they did not need it. I was lead to begin in Matthew and learned about

Jesus. I began to learn His ways and see His compassion. I had to repent and ask God for forgiveness. You know I was told a lot of things about Jesus, which are false. I use to role with a reading group that really had it in for Him. They use to call Him, J. C. and joke about Him and say all sorts of terrible things about Him. Remember, I was going to church every Sunday, and I sat and listened to that trash about the God I professed to serve. What, did I look like to them? **What do we** look like to the world?

The real problem was, **I was not reading my bible.** I was **too lazy** and I allowed the preacher and who ever to tell me about Jesus. I, until that day, had not sort a relationship for myself, it was all here say. So, when people told lies about Jesus, I did not even know if they were right or wrong. I felt funny being there, but I had no ammunition against the attack. The Bible says, ***"My people are destroyed for lack of knowledge."*** I was truly, dying daily for lack of knowledge. The crazy thing was, I did not have the **sense**, to go and research for myself, to see if what they said was true. I was bound by ignorance.

When I began to read, I got to know Jesus. Jesus allowed me to see myself in Him. Soon He started to reveal to me all that I had done in my life against Him. All the hours of abuse I suffered for lack of knowledge. He told me about my relationship with Al and the choices I made to perpetuate it. He made me stop focusing on just blaming Al, and look at me. He was cleansing me with the blood. At first I cried a lot and I prayed. Then, I repented to God, and everything changed.

The sister had a clock in her home, and that clock rang at prayer time. So whenever it rang, I would pray. Then, when I would read, He would show me something else. After all the sin was gone, He started to show me some of the benefits of having a relationship with God. He began showing me how I should live. And how that life could bring joy, peace and forgiveness. Forgiveness for me, Al and all the people who had hurt me and took advantage of me over the years. I felt great. God had given me salvation as a free gift. Since His Son had paid the price and redeemed me from sin. Then, one day I realized, that by being obedient to His word, I had accepted Him as Lord of my life. Hallelujah! Hallelujah! Hallelujah! I am free. And those that the Son sets free are free indeed.

My salvation took place at home so, He led me to become a member of a church with an anointed man of God as head. A man seeking understanding and revelation from God; who is the source of all things. After about three months of straight study, I had to leave my friend's home. She was getting back together with her husband. That was cool; the time I needed to build a relationship with my Lord was done.

I am eternally grateful to God for using her and to Pam for her obedience to come and offer me a place to stay. I thank and praise God for sending His Spirit to teach me about His Word. I thank and praise Him in advance for all that will be touched by these words and begin a journey toward Jesus. I thank Him for the ones who will see that church attendance is not enough, any more and seek a deeper walk with God. I praise Him for the ones who will have the guts to come out of the shallow waters and go into the deep.

If your reading this book and have not Accepted God's invitation to His Son Christ Jesus and been saved. Or are not sure what it means, I would like to ask you a few questions. Think about where you are right now in your life... Are you unhappy with where you are? Is your future dim or uncertain? Have you been searching for something, not being able to put your finger on just what it is? Do you know you need to change, but don't know how? If you have answered yes to one or all of the proceeding questions, let me ask you a few more... Do you want a relationship with God? If yes, continue. Do you know that you are a sinner? Will you ask God for forgiveness of those sins? Do you believe Jesus is the

Son of God? Do you believe that He died on the cross for your sins and arose again on the third day? Now that you have read the words, do you believe them? Are you willing to say them out loud to someone else? If you answered yes to the last two questions, according to Romans 10:9 you are saved. Hallelujah! Hallelujah! Hallelujah! Welcome to the family of God.

God freely gives salvation to those He purposed from the foundation of the world. And if you have answered truthfully, He is pleased to send His spirit into your heart. You don't work for salvation it's a gift. You should feel really good right now, but you will need to pick up your armor ***(Ref. Ephesians 6:10-18)*** and put it on, that you will be able to stand in the army of the Lord of Host, Jehovah Sabboath. Let us look to God.

Father, I ask you right now, in the Name of Jesus: Renew a right spirit within each one of the readers today. Pique their interest to want to know you better. Allow your Spirit to stir up in them a renewed hunger and thirst for your word, which can only be quenched by being in your presence. We recognize that man cannot live by bread alone, but by every word that proceeds out of the mouth of God. Lord, we thank you that your word is a lamp unto our feet and a light unto our path. God, we ask that you order our steps in your word. Lord, lead us on the straight and narrow path that leads to life. We thank and praise you for your Word, that directs us and Your Spirit that guides us into Your Truth, all these things we ask you for and thank you for, in Jesus' Name. Amen.

To God Be The Glory!!!

Please complete this form before you proceed with the book.

1. How often do you go to church? ______________________

2. Are you born again? _____________

3. Would you like to be? __________ Or Are you living for Jesus? ___________

    a. Jesus gives us direction to heaven…John 3:3
    b. Where do we start?…Romans 3:23
    c. God gives the answer…Romans 6:23
    d. God shows His great love for us…Romans 5:8
    e. Jesus shows us the way…John 14:6
    f. Now that you know something about the Heart of God can Confess what you know…Rom.10:9
    g. Commit to a bible study to grow in Him…Matt 11:25-30
    h. What's the other alternative…1 Corinthians 6:9-11

The Prayer:

Father, I come before you as your child asking your forgiveness. I ask that You forgive me of my sins and cleanse me from all unrighteousness, as you promised. I know that Jesus is the Way, the Truth and the Life and the only way that I may have an opportunity to see You is by Him. Father, help me to accept the righteousness that you have made me that I will look and act like Jesus. So, Father please, examine me, and know my heart, test me and know my thoughts. See if there is any hurtful, wicked or deceitful way in me and lead me in the way of everlasting. Order my steps in your word, that I may know your goodness, mercy, truth, forgiveness, power and love. And stand in my rightful place as Son/Daughter of God. All these things I ask in Jesus' Name. Amen.

Name: ____

Address: ______________________________________

____

Commitment Bible study: ________________________________

Seek God-Where He can be found

The word of God calls us to ***study to show thy self approved unto God, a workman that needs not to be ashamed rightly dividing the words of truth (II Timothy 2:15).KJV*** Before you got saved you lived a life that you thought was correct. A life based solely on the world's system. A system that has no communion with God. The word of God lets us know that, ***the natural man cannot understand the ways of God.*** Now is the time to begin your education in God's system of things. Don't look at what you see people doing to find your way. The Bible says, the majority of people are outside the will of God.

Jesus said, *"Enter ye in at the strait gate: for wide is the gate, and broad is the way, that leadeth to destruction, and many there be which go in thereat: Because strait is the gate, and narrow is the way, which leadeth unto life, and few there'll be that find it." Matthew 7:13-14*

Remember that group includes people who go to church every Sunday. Knowing that, lets look to God. Dear heavenly Father, We thank you that you are God and none stands by you. That you are Alpha and Omega, The Beginning and The Ending. We recognize that by your word, you created the world and all living creatures there in. So, Father as we seek you where you can be found, in your word. We ask that you Search us, O God and know our hearts: try us, and know our thoughts: and see if there be any wicked way in us. And led us in the way everlasting. In Jesus' Name. Amen. (Psalms139:23-24).

[The following are a few scriptures to help you on your way towards building a relationship with God. Remember, it does not matter where you begin, just as long as you begin reading the word on a daily basis.]

I. Matthew

II. Luke

III. John

IV. Romans

V. Philippians

VI. James

VII. Galatians

VIII. Ephesians

IX. I, II & III John

Please take as much time as you need with each chapter to allow God to reveal His Word to you. Look for yourself in the word. Be obedient to the word. When God starts to deal with you about something, **you'll need to either put it down or pick it up.** Please, don't fight. Your under His grace **for a time**, but don't test God. If you do, you won't receive the life His Son died for you to have, because you have chosen to be a worker of iniquity. There is a difference in being a sinner and worker of iniquity.

To be clear, a sinner- one who is on the outside of God's word. One who has not accepted Jesus Christ as their Lord and Savior. They practice sin and their sins in this world are upon them. You see when you accepted Jesus as your Lord and Savior, your sins were cleansed by the blood of Jesus. You were made the righteousness of God, when Jesus was made sin for you. If you sin, your not a sinner, you are still the righteousness of God. Although, God expects you to repent **immediately** and **continue in your righteousness.** Remember, the righteousness of God practice righteousness. Don't allow guilt and depression to keep you from the presence of God. He knows you.

Now, if you sin and continue in sin, since you think you are covered by grace, you make a mockery of the Blood of Jesus. So, then you are counted as a worker of iniquity. Remember, Jesus saved you from sin. So, why would you even think that you are suppose to continue to act like the sinful world? ***Shall we continue in sin that grace may abound? God Forbid.*** Reading, studying and obeying His word will make you a new creature in Christ Jesus. ***Romans 12:1-2 states, I beseech you therefore, brethren, by the mercies of God, that ye present your bodies a living sacrifice, holy, acceptable unto God,*** *which is your reasonable service. And be not conformed to this world: but be ye transformed by the renewing of your mind, that ye may prove what is that good, and acceptable, and perfect, will of God.*

Jesus said, *"Beware of false prophets, which come to you in sheep's clothing, but inwardly they are ravening wolves. Ye shall know them by their fruits. Do men gather grapes of thorns, or figs of thistles? Even so every good tree brings forth good fruit; but a corrupt tree brings forth evil fruit. A good tree cannot bring forth evil fruit; neither can a corrupt tree bring forth good fruit. Every tree that brings not forth good fruit is hewn down, and cast into the fire. (Hell) Wherefore by their fruits ye shall know them. Not every one that saith unto me, Lord, Lord, shall enter into the kingdom of heaven; but he that doeth the will of my Father which is in heaven. Many will say to Me in that day, Lord, Lord, have we not prophesied in thy name? And in thy name have cast out devils? And in thy name done many wonderful works? And then will I profess unto them, I never knew you: depart from me, ye that work iniquity. Matthew 7:15-23*

God protects us and says, nothing can take us from His hands. But if we willingly get out from under, the ark of safety, and go on our own way, serving Satan or becoming our own god, that's idolatry. Idolaters have no place in the kingdom of God.

I Corinthians 6:9-11 Know ye not that the unrighteous shall not inherit the kingdom of God? Be not deceived: neither fornicators, nor idolaters, nor adulterers, nor effeminate, nor abusers of themselves with mankind. Nor thieves, nor covetous, nor drunkard, nor revilers, nor extortioners, shall inherit the kingdom of God. And such were some of you: but ye are washed, but ye are sanctified, but ye are justified in the name of the Lord Jesus, and by the Spirit of your God.

Hold fast to the confession of your faith. Don't allow a non-believer to change your mind. They have no clue about what God is about to do in your life. ***Only be thou strong and very courageous, that thou mayest*** *observe to do according to all the law, which Moses my servant commanded thee: turn not from it to the right hand or to the left, that thou mayest prosper whithersoever thou goest. This book of the law shall not depart out to thy mouth; but thou shalt meditate therein day and night, that thou mayest observe to do according to all that is written therein: for then thou shalt make thy way prosperous, and then thou shalt have good success. Joshua 1:7-8*

Please, take the time to read, study and meditate on the scriptures above. Without being led by the spirit and having a relationship with God, there is no way the rest of the book will make any sense to you. The natural man cannot understand the things of God. Lose your mind and put on the mind of Christ, that you may be able to see, hear, experience and find Him early when you seek Him.

If You Love Me Keep My Commandments...John 14:15

1. Thou shall not have no other gods before Me.

Any thing that you want to do that takes up your prearranged time with God is a small-g god in your life. If you watch football, play baseball, soccer, basketball, wash your car, go shopping, sleep, work, etc., you have made that thing, a god, and that's idolatry. That does not only include Sunday church service. Anything during prayer service, bible study, your prayer time or Sunday school, our Bible says that we are not to forsake the fellowship of the saints. If you are already in that situation, and you just got saved, trust God and follow His leadership. God will instruct you in His Word, He will lead you to the church that He wants you to go to and provide a way for you to make it there.

2.. Thou shall not make unto thee any graven images; thou shall not bow down thy self to them.

For far to many years the image of Michael Angelo has been in the minds, on the walls, on the church bulletin, on church fans, in stain glass, on billboards and on television for all to see. That lie has gone on long enough. There are no actual recorded pictures of Jesus. Nowhere in the scriptures did it say that while on their way to

Jerusalem, Jesus and the disciples, stopped to pose for a portrait. Nor do the scriptures allege that there was a painter among the people that gathered for the last supper. The bible has to be the first and last authority in our lives. ***Study to show thy self approved of God, a workman that needs not to be ashamed, rightly dividing the word of truth.***

2 Timothy 2:15

3. Thou shall not take the name of the Lord thy God in vain.

When you accepted God's invitation to Christ and became saved, it was the most joyous day in heaven. You had come out of the darkness into the marvelous light. While your were in darkness you did things that promoted darkness and the prince of that world. Now that you have become Christ's, you put away the old things and behold all things have become new. You are a new creature. Now, to live the way God wants you to live, you have to be re-educated in the ways of God. Salvation is instant, but sanctification is a process. Sanctification is the process of putting down the ways of the world and picking up the ways of God and learning to walk in that new lifestyle. It takes time but you can do it.

All of the old things won't just go away instantly. As you stay in the word, you will, slowly or quickly, (depending on how diligent your study is), find out all the things that are wrong with you that need to be changed. It is going to be ruff, depending on your age and willingness to change. The more willing you are, the less pain, but the less willing the greater the pain you will suffer. If you study, on your own, The Holy Spirit will teach you and you won't be embarrassed in front of people. BUT IF YOU REFUSE, to be taught by The Holy Spirit, you open yourself up, to be taught by others. People, even other Christians don't have the same great Love and Compassion that God has. So, save yourself some additional pain and suffering by being taught by God through His Word. Then you can **stand** (producing meekness and long suffering) and be the Christian that you were saved to be. Not taking God's name in vain.

Let me explain something to you, when you continue in sin your salvation is in question. Were you serious when you said you loved God and believed that Jesus died for you? Or were you just playing to get into the club? God knows the heart of a man (woman). You may, be able to fool some of the people, some of the time or all of the people most of time, but you will **never** be able to fool God, ever. ***Not every one that saith unto me, Lord, Lord, shall enter into the kingdom of heaven; but he that doeth the will of my Father which is in heaven. Many will say to me in that day, Lord, Lord, have we not*** *prophesied in they name? And in thy name have cast out devils? And in thy name done many wonderful works? And then will I profess unto them, I never knew you: depart from me, ye that work iniquity. Matthew 7:21-23*

Walking in His word will keep you form taking His name in vain. His name is Holy. His name is pure. His name is righteous. **People are watching you.** Be the salt, that you were saved to be so, that your life can be an example to all those who are watching you. If your going to play with God and do your own thing, you might as well stop going to church. You give real Christians a bad name by meeting the unsaved in the bar Saturday night and the saints in church Sunday morning. God is watching you and you will pay for mis-representing His name.

Romans 8: 6-10 For to be carnally minded is death; but to be spiritually minded is life and peace. Because the carnal mind is enmity against God: for it is not subject to the law of God, neither indeed can be. So, then they that are in the flesh cannot please God. But ye are not in the flesh, but in the spirit, if so be that the Spirit of God dwell in you. Now, if any man have not the Spirit of Christ, he is none of His. And if Christ be in you, the body is dead because of sin; but the Spirit is life because of righteousness.

4. Remember the Sabbath day to keep it Holy.

There are seven days in the week, six to work and worship and the other for worship, fellowship and thanksgiving to God. A day where God will be praised for the glory He has done in you, that you could not do for yourself. God is saying to us, "You Better Recognize." Salvation is of God, and **God alone**. So, give Him the Praise and Glory for what He has done. He purposed it in the beginning, that we might remember that God is our Salvation, and none stands by Him. There is no amount of work that you could ever do to save yourself. It's a gift so, just receive it.

Now, if you are thinking, I have to work seven days a week, to keep my house or apartment. Your house is too expensive and you have been an unprofitable steward of God's money. Now, you have become an idolater since you have put that house in front of God. If your saying to yourself, I have to work seven days a week to pay my car note. You have placed that car in God's first place status and you are an idolater. My children need better or more clothes, I want to go on vacation, I need to get my hair and nails done or what ever it is that you are trying to get, instead of a closer walk with God, has become the **god** in your life.

If you want more money, sow your tithes an offering. God says, ***"Prove me now here with, If I will not open you the windows of heaven, and pour you out a blessing, that there shall not be room enough to receive it." Malachi 3:10b*** Anytime you take money out of God's house for your own selfish needs, you cut a whole in your pocket that will leave you always in need of more. The only way you will be prosperous is to obey God's voice and keep His charge, commandments, statues and laws. ***James 4:2-4 states, Ye lust, and have not: ye kill, and desire to have, and cannot obtain: ye fight and war, yet ye have not. Because ye ask not. Ye ask, and receive not, because ye ask amiss. That ye may consume it upon***

your lusts. Ye adulterers and adulteresses, know ye not that the friendship of the world is enmity with God? Whosoever therefore will be a friend of the world is the enemy of God.

5. Honor thy Father and Mother; that thy days be long upon the land in which the lord thy God giveth thee.

Mom and Dad have been here many years longer than you. We pray to God that they have been walking in God's word. Amen. Therefore, their counsel is for your benefit, health, safety, guidance, comfort and keeping.

Parents keep in mind that this commandment assumes that you are obeying God's voice and passing His

teachings down to your children. When you don't obey, then you move into the realm where Paul says, ***Fathers provoke not your children to wrath, but bring them up in the nurture and admonition of the Lord. Ephesians 6:4*** The quickest way to bring your child to wrath is for you to live contradictory to your own teachings. Children today will do, not what you say, but what you do, and then remind you of what you do, to back up their claim to unrighteousness. So, parents train up a child in the way they should go, by **God's word, your words and your actions.**

Children, while you were young they (your parents), took care of you, but when you become an adult and they are in their golden years, you will need to honor them in a financial way also. You should not be using your Father and Mother as your personal ATM machine. Jesus rebuked the religious leaders for keeping a tradition, instead of God's command. By allowing people to use the money for their parents, for alms or church contributions for profit, thereby, releasing them from their responsibility of honoring their parents. Ref. Matthew 15:1-8 Don't take up traditions that contradict God's Word. ***Heaven and earth shall pass away, but My Words shall never pass away. Matthew 24:35 Fear not them which kill the body, but are not able to kill the soul: but rather***

fear Him which is able to destroy both soul and body in hell. Matthew 10:28

6. Thou shall not kill.

Of course we know that shooting, stabbing, strangling, drowning, bleeding, poisoning, abortion and a host of other cruel and indecent acts will suspend life. Now, lets talk about the blood less deaths that occur without our conscience. We are commanded to love our brother, neighbors and enemies. If love is pro-life then to hate would be anti-life. So, how do we kill without blood shed? ***Matthew 5:21-22 states, You have heard that it was said to the people long ago; Do not murder and anyone***

who murders will be subject to judgment but, I tell you that anyone who is angry with his brother will be subject to judgment, Again anyone who says to his brother Raca is answerable to the Sanhedrin (counsel).NKJV Now Raca means empty or worthless. Now-a-days we here people say, "Shut up!, Stupid!", "Dummy," and "You're like a brick wall" "You'll never amount to anything" or "Your just like your no-good father" or some other vile remark. Please have mercy on our children.

Our text talks about speaking this way to your brother but many of our parents speak this way to their children. Can a mother kill her child? Yes! With words that have a sting that will last longer than any blow of belts or switches. I believe all of the car thieves, drug dealers, muggers and other social paths had contradiction in their lives. Parents provoke not your children to wrath.

7. Thou shall not commit adultery.

We all know that the relationship between, "Me and Mrs. Jones" is adultery but, what about the stop me in my tracks looks, that I give to Mrs. Robinson or Tara Banks. OOH! the thoughts that go through my mind, Um, Um, Um. What I could do if I had a woman like that. Or ladies, what about Mr. Robinson or Denzel Washington, tall, dark, handsome and bulky in all the right places. How far do our minds wonder before we catch them? We need to know that, ***the weapons of our warfare are not carnal, but mighty through God to the pulling down of strong holds; Casting down imaginations and every high thing that exalts it self against the knowledge of God, bringing into captivity every thought to the obedience of Christ. 2 Corinthians 10:4-5.*** If you don't do that, all those lustful thoughts will kill you. ***Matthew 5:27-28 Ye have heard that it was said by them of old time, thou shalt not commit adultery: But I say unto you, that whosoever looks at a woman/man to lust after her/him hath committed adultery with her/him already in his/her heart.***

8. Thou shalt not steal.

The first thing we think of is armed robbery of banks, corner stores, people in the street at night and unsuspecting motorist on that lonely, dark street at the light. Theft has many more realms to it then commonly discussed. The main one ***Malachi 3:8- 9 Will a man rob God? Yet ye have robbed Me. But ye say, wherein have we robbed thee? In tithes and offering. You are under a curse the whole nation of you because you are robbing Me. Bring the whole tithe into the store house, that there may be food in My house. Test Me in this, says the Lord Almighty and see if I will not open you the windows of***

heaven, an pour you out a blessing, that you will not have room enough to receive it.

If you decide **not** to taste and see, that the Lord is good, and settle for not enough or just enough, below what God has for you and not tithe; ***Know that the wicked will not inherit the Kingdom of God? Do not be deceived: neither the sexually immoral nor idolaters nor adulterers nor male prostitutes nor homosexual offenders nor thieves nor the greedy nor drunkards nor slanderers nor swindlers will inherit the Kingdom of God. 1Corinthians 6:9-10 niv*** Remember, God said **bring** the **tithe**, He did not say, **If you want to prosper**, this is what you do. Obedience is better than sacrifice.

9. Thou shalt not bear false witness against thy neighbor.

We know that half truth, part truth, wrong context truth, misrepresented truth, distorted truth and left out truth, all add up to one **BIG FAT LIE!!!** Let us not deceive ourselves, Christians. Telling your child to tell a bill collector, your girlfriend, your mother, your sister or brother in Christ, that you are not at home, is a lie from the pit. When we begin to accept responsibility for our tongues, actions and acted upon thoughts we will all be better off. Then we will be able to allow God to do the work He wants to do in our lives.

Why do we lie? We think we lie to protect others, For instance your girl friend has on an ugly hat that should have stayed on the rummage sale table. She asks you. "How do you like it?" You lie and say, "You go girl, that hat is smokin'," all the while your thinking, burning in a bone fire would be better. You did not lie to protect her, you lied to protect yourself from honesty. All you had to say was, If you like it, that's fine but, its not my style of hats. Or you could tell her straight, the hat is not pretty, nor flattering to you, your face, your outfit or what ever the situation is. Your friend will accept or reject your opinion anyway, but you would not have added one more sin, to your stack that you forgot to repent for.

On the other hand if your friend asks your advice about something that is contrary to God's word. Please don't allow **fear** to cause you to sin against God. If your buddy says, "Man I'm going to get that girl right over there. I'm going to wine her, dine her and have my way with her." Don't stand there looking all amazed and happy with his intent. Stand up and be the man that you say you are, and tell the truth. Please, don't try to hide behind other excuses why he should not do it like; She looks dirty. He'll just say, "I have protection". She's not that cute. He'll say, "She will be when the lights are off."

Why not wait? "There is no time like the present." There is no way to get out of a sticky situation than with God's honest truth. Listen man, I would not if I were you. My relationship with God is too important to give up for one night of passion, that won't live up to the expectation. ***1 Corinthians 6:18 says, Flee fornication, every sin that a man does is without the body; but he that commit fornication sins against his own body. What? Know ye that your body is the temple of the Holy Ghost, which is in you, which ye have of God, and ye are not your own? For ye are bought with a price: Therefore, glorify God in your body, and in your spirit which are God's.***

10. Thou shall not covet thy neighbors house, wife, servants, animals or any thing that belongs to thy neighbor.

The most common form of coveting, would be to try to keep up with the Jones. Always thinking that "The grass is greener on the other side of the fence." If you get to work on your **own yard**, your **own wife**, your **own children**, your **own car**, your **own Church**, your **own tongue**, your **own walk with God**, your **own study time**, your **own prayer life**, your **own tithing**, your **own witnessing** and **coveting your own gifts of the spirit**, then God will bless you to have. He promises to prosper you in whatsoever you do.

Be not deceived; God is not mocked: for whatsoever a man sows, that shall he also reap. For he that sows to his flesh shall of the flesh reap corruption; but he that Sows to the Spirit shall of the Spirit reap life everlasting. And let us not be weary in well doing: for in due season we shall reap, if we faint not. Galatians 6:7-9 But seek ye first the Kingdom of God, and His righteousness; and all these things shall be added unto you. Take therefore no thought for the morrow; for the morrow shall take thought for the things of itself. Sufficient unto the day is the evil thereof. Matthew 6: 33-34

Hold fast to all the commandments and the promises that are yea and Amen, to the obedient ones. No one is perfect but, we are striving for perfection in the eyes of God. So, let us repent; Dear Heavenly Father, I had no idea my ways contradicted you this much. I have adopted these habits out of ignorance. Please forgive me for the trust-pass and lead me on the path of righteousness for your Name sake. In Jesus Name, Amen. Now, be ready to do things the right way. Set your mind to be aware of your actions. Please don't beat yourself up every time you mess up. Just repent(ask God for forgiveness and turn from the path that takes you to that sin). Then, continue in righteousness. You'll get the hang of it real soon.

Know your rights against the devil and his demons. Don't be afraid of them. Know that Jesus has sent His Spirit to give us *the power to tread upon serpents and scorpions, and over all of the power of the enemy and nothing shall by any means hurt you. Luke 10:19. Who shall separate us from the love of Christ: Shall tribulation, or distress, or persecution, or famine, or nakedness, or peril or sword? As it is written for thy sake we are killed all the day long; we are accounted as sheep for the slaughter. Nay, in all these things we are more than conquerors through Him that loved us. For I am persuaded that neither death, nor life, nor angel, nor principality, nor powers, nor things present, nor things to come, nor height, nor depth, nor any other creature, shall be able to separate us from the love of God, which is in Christ Jesus our Lord. Romans 8:35-39 Amen. To God Be The Glory.*

Ask and ye shall receive

God has so many promises within the bible that are ye and Amen, that no one should go without answers to their prayers. God's promises covers everything from health to wealth, promotion to longevity, defeat of the enemy to rebuke of the devourer. So, why do prayers go unanswered? Well, I know if God said it, He meant it and He can, will and watches over His word to perform it. So, what's the problem? **Instability**. People won't stay faithful to God long enough for God to bring His word to pass in their lives. The word says, ***"If you <u>abide</u> in me and my word abides in you, ask what you will and it shall***

be done unto you. Jn15:7" So, even if you ask for a million dollars, God will give it. Remember God cannot be wasteful so, He will have to prepare you to receive it first. That's the main reason for the delay. Now, if you start talking against your prosperity or eat your seeds for harvest, you won't receive the prayer request.

That's the point that Satan comes in and says, see I knew that prayer stuff did not work, then you think, I'll do it my self next time. Just a little doubt will kill your belief in God and make you an idolater. Remember, God's promises are sure. If you have not received, the problem will ALWAYS be with you NOT GOD. Have patience and wait for God. Know ahead of time that you will experience some trouble and look forward to it. Change your mind about it and you will withstand it every time. ***James 1:2 -8 says, My brethren, count it all joy when ye fall into divers temptations; knowing this that the trying of your faith works patience. But let patience have her perfect work, that ye may be perfect and entire, wanting nothing. If any of you lack wisdom, let him ask of God, that gives to all men liberally, and upbraideth not. And it shall be given him. <u>But let him ask in faith nothing wavering, for he that wavers is like a wave of the sea driven with the wind and tossed, For let not that man think that he shall receive any thing of the Lord.</u> A double minded man is unstable in all his ways.***

Obedience to the word of God is another way for God to move on your behalf. Whatever your asking God to do in your life, you must be prepared to do the same for others. The word says, if you want a friend, show yourself friendly. Do unto others as you will have them do unto you. **You do first.** If you want money, give money. ***Be not deceived; God is not mocked: for whatsoever a man sows, that, shall he also reap. Galatians 5:7*** Don't sow peach seeds if you want watermelon. Now, if you have a request, other than money, you can allow your willingness to sow against, **the root of evil**(love of money), for the amplification of your request. Say you want a friend, you can show yourself friendly and give toward the benevolence offering as a memorial seed. Be willing to give more than just a prayer or time into peoples lives. That's how you stand out from the crowd. Now remember, your not giving it to be seen, or you will have your reward. God sees all things done in secret and rewards you openly.

Now back to the million dollars. The first thing you will need to do is sow your tithes regularly. If you were not, repent to God for the theft, make a commitment and stick to it. If you cannot be trusted to sow tithes for $10 how will God ever be able to trust you with a $1M dollars? Keep in mind none of it belongs to you. You are a steward of God's money. Think to yourself, I will need to do on command whatever He says to do with it. It's easier, to give someone else things, than it is to give yours. Your obedience will lead to increase. If what you have in your hand does not meet your need, it's a seed. So, ***Give and it shall be given unto you; good measure, pressed down, and shaken together, and running over, shall men give unto you bosom, For with the same measure that ye mete with it shall be measured to you again. (Luke 6:38)*** When the increase comes, put it back into the ground until its your desired harvest. Be ready for whenever and whatever God tells you to give. God does not mind you having plenty of money, houses, cars, jewelry or any of the things of this world. He just wants you to keep them in the right perspective. ***Seek ye first the kingdom of God and His righteousness; and all these things shall be added unto you. Matthew 6:33***

God wants to do, what He said he would do, in your life. So, don't make up a scenario and try to get God to go along with what you want. Remember God said in ***Isaiah 55:8-11, For My thoughts are not your thoughts, neither are your ways My ways, saith the Lord. For as the heavens are higher than the earth, so are My ways higher than your way, and My thoughts than your thoughts, For as the rain cometh down, and snow from heaven, and returneth not thither, but watereth the earth, and maketh it bring forth and bud, that it may give seed to the*** *sower, and bread to the eater: So shall My Word be that goeth forth out of My mouth: it shall not return unto Me void, but it shall accomplish that which I please, and it shall prosper in the thing where to I sent it.* God has only promised to bring His word to pass. So, you must seek God for your solution, then, in your prayers ask for what He has promised.

Now, don't think you can serve Satan and beg God. When God speaks to you, you must answer yes, Amen and I will do it. *Be ye a doer of the word and not a hearer only deceiving yourself. James 1:22* Please, don't try to 'fake it,' to get what you want from Him. God knows a mans heart. You cannot trick Him. If you try, you will feel the wrath of God. ***Be not deceived God is not mocked: whatsoever a man sows, that shall he also reap, For he that sows to his flesh shall of the flesh reap corruption; but he that sows to the Spirit shall of the Spirit reap life everlasting. Galatians 6:7-8***

Decide for yourself that serving Satan has gotten you no-where. Decide right now to change. Allow God to cleanse you so, that you can ask for what you want and get it. Jesus confirms that in ***John 15:1-7, I am the true vine, and my Father is the husbandman. Every branch in Me that beareth not fruit he taketh away: and every branch that beareth fruit, he purgeth it, that it may bring forth more fruit. Now ye are clean through the word*** *which I have spoken unto you. Abide in me, and I in you as the branch cannot bear fruit of itself, except it abide in the vine; no more can ye except you abide in me. I am the vine, ye are the branches. He that abideth in me, and I in him, the same bringeth forth much fruit: <u>for without Me ye can do nothing.</u> If a man abide not in me, he is cast forth as a branch, and is withered; and men gather them, and cast them into the fire, and they are burned. <u>If ye abide in me and my words abide in you, ye shall ask what ye will, and it shall be done unto you.</u>*

God is not a man that He should lie. When He says something, it shall be done. God's words are not by chance, luck or only for some people. God has a system of principles set up from the beginning of time. Anyone who gets involved with them and has the guts to believe God, can have some marvelous things happen for them. I have personally asked God for something and gotten it in a matter of hours. It did not look like what I asked for at first so, I resisted a bit. Then, the Spirit told me not to resist or disobey authority. So, the place I did not want to go ended up being the place where my blessing was. Gods thoughts are truly not our thought and His ways are not our ways. So, when you ask Him for something, watch out! How you act and how you treat people. Since, you don't know where your blessing is going to come from. God has a way of blessing you and teaching you something at the same time. He is so, Awesome, and Wonderful and Unique and All Knowing that you will not be able to deny that it was Him that blessed you. So, I suppose the prayer that follows the request would be, (mostly to prepare your mind), Father God, give it to me anyway you like and I will be satisfied. In Jesus' Name. Amen. Pray in the Holy Ghost. **Then trust God and do good.** Your answer is on the way. Please don't doubt and for your harvest sake, don't speak against it. If you find yourself with nothing to do, praise God(Jehovah Jireh), for what He has already done, and sow your best seed offering, for your harvest is on the way.

That's the Super now the natural. As you pray in the Spirit (Pray in tongues) The Holy Spirit is digging into the things of God that can lead you into profit. You are calling up wisdom that will reveal to you the path that you should take to acquire the wealth. God is not just going to give it to you in the mail. You will have to work hard to develop the idea that God gave you to generate your millions. You see the Spirit can give you ideas and witty inventions that if you develop them God will cause people to need your invention or idea.

What is it inside of you that God has showed you to do that you have neglected for lack of self esteem or for fear of ridicule? To get to your wealthy place your going to have to step out on some of those ideas and trust God to see you through. What if I miss it? Well sometimes you have to miss it to make it. Start on a road, then when you see its not the one then, you can turn, but don't just stand there. The Holy Spirit is a helper not an initiator. He will help you in what you do. He will never do for you **what you can do.** Sure, He is there to do what you can't do and pray what you don't know and lead you where you thought you could not go, but <u>He will not do your part also.</u>

Faith operates everything in the Kingdom of God and fear operates everything of the devil. Knowing that, even if your afraid step out to do what the Holy Spirit is saying you can do. You take a step and He is right there with you. Take me for instance. I never in a million years thought of being a writer. I know I had a passion to help people see that every answer to every situation in life is in the Bible. That God is the creator and He has to know more than we so, why not seek His face for answers to our problems and get the solution that will benefit for eternity.

Even when I was not saved, I knew that God was greater than me. I did not know a fraction of what I know now but, I still had since enough to know what minute understanding I have now, is less than one nanometer of ½ less than one fraction of a mustard grain of knowledge compared to God's infinite wisdom. I am in awe of Him, and all that He has taught me, through Him giving me the wisdom, to write this manuscript. Jesus is my All and All. He is everything and without Him I am nothing. God gets all of the Praise and Honor and Glory for what He has done in my life. I am grateful that He allowed me to aid in the spread of His word.

So, what is driving you? What idea is burning in your heart? What has God already showed you that you can do? What do you have in your house? Get it and seek God for His wisdom in how to develop it into a marketable product or service. ***Ask, and it shall be given you; seek, and ye shall find; knock, and it shall be***

opened unto you: For every one that asketh receivethe; and he that seeketh findeth; and to him that knocketh it shall be opened. Mt 7:7-8 God is ready to do some awesome things in these last days so, repent to God and become what He created you to be. Then you will truly see how effective your prayers will become.

Train up a child

Our heavenly Father has entrusted parents with the gift of children. It is the parents responsibility to guild, protect and bring them up in the nurture and the admonition of the Lord. To truly be effective in this task, you must embody the principles that have been given to us by our heavenly Father. He is the first father and He created parenthood so, trust that He knows something about the task before you.

Remember, in training up a child, the training is not only by your words, but the follow up is your actions. If you tell your child not to lie, you must speak the truth. If you want your child to have love and respect for authority, you must first respect the authority of God, your church leaders and your parents. Children learn better by example. If you want your child to be better than you, you must give them a better example in the form of Jesus Christ the perfect example of humanity. Lead them in the way that they should go so, when the world offers them heartaches and misfortunes they can have the solid rock to stand on, that the gates of hell will not prevail against them.

Sunday School is a great place to reinforce the values you have already instilled in your children. The word of God in their lives will lead them on the road to excellence and increase in their lives. Your children will learn very important skills that will help them be productive members in church, school and society in general. They will learn God's way of handling problems and situations before they get into them. Every child should experience the love of God so, that he will have that love in his heart for those around him.

In Sunday School the basic setup is this; Study the lesson at home before you get to class. In class read and review all questions and points. Then, the class works out some real life applications to make the lesson real. Finally, the class stands before the entire Sunday School to give an oral report of what was learned and how it effects the lives of the students today.

Study before class will help your children be prepared for any situation they will encounter in the future. It may be higher learning, a career or owning their own business, but preparation is needed for all. In class reading shows them that there is a time to speak, and a time listen, a time to do, and a time wait, a time to be creative, and a time to follow directions. We learn that there is a time and place for everything and to learn when, where and how to distinguish those times in our lives is very important in being prepared for the moves of God.

We work out life applications because we need to know that life is a continuous cycle of sowing and reaping. We need to learn how to communicate with one another, how to treat one another and to care for one another. We have to learn how to honor God in all our body, mind, soul and lifestyle. We will also learn, to encourage one another and be encouraged by others. We learn to give and take criticism without getting an attitude when someone tells us where we have gone astray. We learn to be convicted by the word, repent and sin no more.

Finally, when we review we learn public speaking. Who knows how many Reverends, politicians, Professors, News reporters, Talk Show host, Teachers, Principals, Hospital

Administrators, CEO's etc., will come out of that Sunday School class. Your children have to be prepared and sanctified, they have to be filled with confidence and the Holy Spirit. They have to know with conviction, "**I can do all things through Christ that strengthens me.**" That first lesson needs to come from people who care about them and love them.

Having a firm foundation in whatever you decide to do, will make your job stress-less and help you to see the pleasure in it. Knowing that God has a purpose for your life, and seeking it while you are young, will help you to have the peace of God that passes all understanding. Then, when you come of age, you will be able to walk in the lifestyle that God has ordained for your life. Knowing your purpose in life will release the pressure of confusion, depression, guilt, despair and pain of trying to figure out why you are on the earth. You will be able to try new things, but not waste time on issues that hinder progress. It will lead you on the road of greatness and increase in your life.

The way we weather storms in our lives is dictated by what we already know about God's word. You cannot see your way through an unforeseen expense unless you know God's a provider. You cannot see your way through a phone call of an accident unless you know God is a protector. You cannot see your way through an illness or disease unless you know God is a healer. You can't see your way through peer pressure, premarital sex, a problem in your marriage, problems at work, depression, loss of relatives, foreclosure on a home, no food in refrigerator or your children in the streets, unless you know God as El Shaddai. The many breasted one, I AM, The One who is more than enough for any situation in your life. Truly Psalms 20:7 says it all, "**Some trust in chariots, and some in horses: but we will remember the name of the Lord our God.**"

In conclusion, our Bible says that we should, "**Train up a child in the way he should go and when he is old he** won't depart from it." Proverb 22:6. Parents you need to know that children will do what you do and often times not what you say. If you are going to raise them in church, have a home lifestyle that compliments and not contradicts the teaching in Sunday School. When you bring your children to church to learn God's way of life and you act like a devil all week long, you are undermining your own child's walk with God. Children need consistency in there life so, that they won't depart from it. When children hear about God and His way of doing things at home, come to church an it's confirmed, visit family members and its reaffirmed, they will be strong in the Lord. Then, when they are faced with negative peer pressure, drugs, premarital sex and/or the wrong crowd, they can stand firm on God's word and not be moved. They will be strong enough to minister to their peers or even become a positive leader in their school's community.

Lack of God's word causes them to lean unto their own understanding. Contradiction makes them say I don't want to go to church. I don't want to be in the Christmas or Easter pageant. Contradiction causes them to rebel against your authority. So, if you are having problems getting your children to listen to you it's because you have to get it together. Repent to God and your children. Then agree, that you all are going to do it God's way. I guarantee, you will have less problems and more love in your happy home.

In Christian Love

Attitude for Increase

To acquire a mind for increase you must first let the mind of Christ be in you so, that you will develop a prosperous spirit. With those thoughts, are forgiveness of sin, healing for your body and soul, deliverance from the guilt of your past, recognition of our covenant, love, power and a sound mind. Once you get a mind like Christ, there will be nothing that can stop you. You will be able to say to that mountain, be ye removed and it will move. Remember, Jesus never let anything stop Him from accomplishing His goal. So, set your mind on the goal to be Christ like and begin to walk that path to eternal life in Christ Jesus. Remember also, life and death is a choice so, let's take God's advice and choose life and meditate on the scriptures that will produce life and increase in every aspect of our lives. Ref. Deuteronomy 30:19

Joshua 1:8 says, "This book of the law shall not depart out of thy mouth; but thou shalt meditate therein day and night, that thou may observe to do according to all that is written therein: for then thou shalt make thy way prosperous and then thou shalt have good success.

Romans 12:1-2 I beseech you therefore, bretheren, by the mercies of God, that ye present your bodies a living sacrifice, holy, acceptable unto God, which is your reasonable service. And be not conformed to this world: but be ye transformed by the renewing of your mind, that ye may prove what is that good, and acceptable, and perfect, will of God.

Psalms 1:1-3 Blessed is the man that walks not in the counsel of the ungodly, nor stands in the way of sinners, nor sits in the seat of the scornful. But his delight is in the law of the Lord; and in his law doth he meditate day and night. And he shall be like a tree planted by the rivers of water, that brings forth his fruit in his season; his leaf also shall not wither; and whatsoever he does shall prosper.

2 Corinthians 10:4-6 For the weapons of our warfare are not carnal, but mighty through God to the pulling down of strong holds; Casting down imaginations, and every high thing that exalts it self against the knowledge of God, and bringing into captivity every thought to the obedience of Christ; And having in a readiness to revenge all disobedience, when your obedience is fulfilled.

Proverbs 4:5-9 Get wisdom, get understanding: forget it not; neither decline from the words of my mouth Forsake her not. And she shall preserve thee: love her, and she shall keep thee. Wisdom is the principal thing; therefore get wisdom: and with all thy getting get understanding. Exalt her, and she shall promote thee: she shall bring thee to honor, when thou dost embrace her. She shall give to thine head an ornament of grace: a crown of glory shall she deliver to thee.

James 1:2-8 My bretheren, count it all joy when ye fall into divers temptations; Knowing this, that the trying of your faith works patience. But let patience have her perfect work, that ye may be perfect and entire, wanting nothing. If any of you lack wisdom, let him ask of God, that giveth to all men liberally, and upbraideth not; and it shall be given him. But let him ask in faith, nothing wavering. For he that wavers is like a wave of the sea driven with the wind and tossed. For let not that man think that he shall receive anything of the Lord. A double minded man is unstable in all his ways.

Daniel 3:16-18 and v24-25 Shadrach, Meshach, and Abednego, answered and said to the king, O Nebuchadnezzar, we are not careful to answer thee in this matter. If it be so, our God whom we serve is able to deliver us out of thine hand, O king. But if not, be it known unto thee, O king, that we will not serve thy gods, nor worship the golden image which thou hast set up. v24-25 Then Nebuchadnezzar the king was astonish, and rose up in haste, and spoke, and said unto his counselors, Did not we cast three men bound into the midst of the fire? They answered and said unto the king, True, O king. He answered and said, Lo, I see four men loose, walking in the midst of the fire, and they have no hurt; and the form of the fourth is like the Son of God.

Proverbs 3:27-35 Withhold not good from them to whom it is due, when it is in the power of thine hand to do it. Say not unto thy neighbor, Go and come again, and tomorrow I will give; when thou hast it by thee. Devise not evil against thy neighbor, seeing he dwells securely by thee. Strive not with a man without cause, if he done thee no harm. Envy thou not the oppressor, and choose none of his ways. For the froward is abomination to the Lord: but His secret is with the righteous. The curse of the Lord is in the house of the wicked: but He blesses the habitation of the just. Surely He scorns the scorners: but He giveth grace unto the lowly. The wise shall inherit glory: but shame shall be the promotion of fools.

1 Thessalonians 5:14-23 Now we exhort you, bretheren, warn them that are unruly, comfort the feebleminded, support the weak, be patient toward all men, See that none render evil for evil unto any man; but ever follow that which is good, both among yourselves, and to all men. Rejoice evermore. Pray without ceasing. In every thing give thanks: for this is the will of God in Christ Jesus concerning you. Quench not the Spirit. Despise not prophesying. Prove all things; hold fast that which is good. Abstain from all appearance of evil and the very God of peace sanctify you wholly; and I pray God your whole spirit and soul and body be preserved blameless unto the coming of our Lord Jesus Christ.

James 4:7-8 Submit yourself therefore to God. Resist the devil, and he will flee from you. Draw nigh to God, and He will draw nigh to you.

Philippians 2: 5-11 <u>Let this mind be in you which is also in Christ Jesus: Who, being in the form of God, thought it not robbery to be equal with God: But made himself of no reputation, and took upon Him the form of a servant, and was made in the likeness of men: and being found in fashion as a man, he humbled himself, and became</u>

obedient unto death, even the death of the cross. Wherefore, God also hath highly exalted him, an given Him name which is above every name: That at the name of Jesus every knee should bow, of things in heaven, and things in earth, and things under the earth; and that every tongue should confess that Jesus Christ is Lord, to the glory of God the Father.

Psalms 119: 11-16 Thy word have I hid in mine heart, that I might not sin against thee. Blessed art thou, O Lord: teach me thy statutes. With my lips have I declared all the judgments of thy mouth. I have rejoiced in the way of thy testimonies, as much as in all riches. I will meditate in *thy precepts, and have respect unto thy ways. I will delight myself in thy statutes: I will not forget thy word.*

John 3:16-17 For God so loved the world, that He gave His only begotten Son, that whosoever believeth in Him should not perish, but have everlasting life. For God sent not His son into the world to condemn the world: but that the world through Him might be saved. He that believeth on Him is not condemned: but he that believeth not is condemned already, because He hath not believed in the name of the only begotten Son of God. And this is the condemnation, that light is come into the world, and men loved darkness rather than light, because their deeds were evil. For every one that does evil hates the light, neither cometh to the light, lest his deeds should be reproved. But he that does truth cometh to the light, that his deeds may be made manifest, that they are wrought in God.

Psalms 100 Make a joyful noise unto the Lord, all ye lands. Serve the Lord with gladness: come before his presence with singing. Know ye that the Lord he is God: it is He that hath made us, and not we ourselves; we are His people, and the sheep of His pasture. Enter into His gates with thanksgiving, and into His courts with praise: be thankful unto Him, and bless His name. For the Lord is good; His mercy is everlasting; and His truth endureth to all generations.

Ephesians 6:10-18 Finally, my bretheren, be strong in the Lord, and in the power of his might. Put on the whole armour of God, that ye may be able to stand against the wiles of the devil. For we wrestle not against flesh and blood, but against principalities, against powers, against the rulers of the darkness of this world, against spiritual wickedness in high places. Wherefore, take unto you the whole armour of God, that ye may be able to withstand in the evil day, and having done all, to stand. Stand, therefore, having your loins girt about with truth, and having on the breastplate of righteousness; and your feet shod with the preparation of the gospel of peace; Above all, taking the shield of faith, wherewith ye shall be able to quench all the fiery darts of the wicked. And take the helmet of salvation, and the sword of the Spirit, which is the Word of God: Praying always with all prayer and supplication in the Spirit, and watching thereunto with all perseverance and supplication for all saints.

When you change your mind about the way you act, talk and treat people to the way God wants you to act, speak and love one another, you will be made into a new creature in Christ Jesus and the gates of hell will not prevail against you. Holiness is accepting God's word and acting on it. Then, you will be walking in the righteousness that the exchange with Jesus has made you. Remember righteous people practice righteousness.

Obedience always comes first so, when you get the increase you will do what God wants you to do with the increase so, that He can increase you more and more. That He may get all the praise and glory. You don't want to get a lump-sum today and be broke again next month. You want to have a continuous flow of resources that increase every time. Now that's what you call the blessings of God. God blesses us to be a blessing to others, **don't ever forget that.** Money always has a mission.

Now there are a few laws that you will need to get involved with to begin the process of increase. The laws are called: Release, Reward, Receiving, Sowing and

Reaping. You will need to **release** to start the process for increase. If you never give, it cannot be given unto you. The word of God says, Whatsoever thou shalt bind on earth shall be bound in heaven; and whatsoever thou shalt loose on earth shall be loosed in heaven. God has already made the laws and it's our responsibility to seek ye first the Kingdom of God, that He can reveal the secrets of the mysteries to us that we may know how to behave in respect to His established principles. Verily, verily I say unto you, Except a corn of wheat fall to the ground and die, it abideth alone: but if it die, it bringeth forth much fruit. Jn12:24 Using the same principle Proverb 11:24-27 says, There is that scattereth, and yet increaseth;

and there is that withholdeth more than is meet, but it tendeth to poverty. The liberal soul shall be made fat: and he that watereth shall be watered also himself. He that withholdeth corn, the people shall curse him: but blessing shall be upon the head of him that selleth it. You'll have to release your time, effort, friendship, and money, that those seeds will sprout a root, that will spring up into your harvest. What more can I say? Obey God.

You will need to work hard to be able to receive a reward for your work. **Doing exactly what God tells you to do will lead you to increase. Don't just look to your regular job for increase from God. Look for the Rhema** word that comes from God. Then work very hard on that so, that you can receive a reward for that. And while at your job, 'Please don't steal time from your boss to do what thus sayeth the Spirit.' Concentrate on, doing more than enough and not just enough. The masses dwell in the just enough, know that its not enough room down there, to spread your wings so, come out from amongst them and fly high. When you get the anointing of excellence on you, you cannot be stopped. Remember to remain meek and humble don't go trying to make people reward you. God sees your work and Jehovah Gomolah will not allow you to work hard and diligent without reward.

Now, when your harvest starts to come forth don't block **some other person's release** for increase by being too self-righteous to **receive** from them. Don't get so caught up in giving that you die from lack. If your giving someone else is receiving so, when your receiving someone else is giving. You must respect the law and allow it to work for everyone around you that wants to participate.

Now, **sowing and reaping** will continue as long as the earth remains. Remember, whatsoever you sow, that you will also reap. So, sow what you want to reap, since you will reap whatever you sow. Understand? It's very simple, please don't try to complicate it with philosophies. If you want a friend, show yourself friendly. If you want to be out of debt, help someone else get out of debt. If you want money, sow money. ***Be not deceived; God is not mocked: for Whatsoever you sow, that you will also reap. Galatians 6:7*** The pressure is not on God it's on your faith to remain faithful and steadfast until your harvest comes. God wants you to have what He promised, but you're the only one that can stop, hinder, remove yourself from the harvesting grounds or block your blessing. God wants to get it to you. Be patient and wait for the Lord. Now wait is not a 'stationary' posture. Isaiah 40:28-31 explains, ***Hast thou not known? Hast thou not heard, that the everlasting God, the Lord,*** *the Creator of the ends of the earth, fainteth not, neither is weary? There is no searching of His understanding. He giveth power to the faint; and to them that have no might he increaseth strength. Even the youths shall faint and be weary, and the young men shall utterly fall: <u>But they that WAIT upon the Lord shall renew their strength; they shall mount up with wings as eagles; they shall run, and not be weary; and they shall walk and not faint</u>.* God does not have to renew the strength of someone who is not doing anything. You're already rested. God renews the strength of His children that have been doing His work. You know the **waiter** in the restaurant, is waiting on tables and people for his employer. Christians serve the people for the Lord. And not just people you know and like, even your enemies that you may be perfect even as your Father is perfect. Then He will sustain you through your journey. To recap: to wait is to serve which equals work. '***Whatsoever He tells you to do, do it.,.***' says, Mary, Mother of Jesus, to the servants.

Remember God is a loving Father. ***Beloved, I wish above all things that you prosper and be in health, even as thy soul prospers. 3Jn2*** God has done an awesome job at giving us the Word (Jesus the perfect example) and His Spirit that will lead us into all truth. Allow the Spirit of God to guide you in this great task. Read and pray every day. Stay in the presence of God that you may find the Way that leads to His will for your life. Remember, the attitude for increase all begins with a choice. ***You, choose life that you and your seed may live.***

Confessions: To the Almighty God

God is my source. The True Vine. He is the Author and Finisher of my faith. He is Alpha and Omega the Beginning and the End. My Bridge over troubled waters. The Bright and Morning Star. The Almighty God, who is more than enough to meet all of our needs. He is the all Knowing. He is ever Present. He is all Powerful. He is Awesome. He is Wonderful. He is Glorious. He is Magnificent. He is Excellent. He is more than I have the words to describe. He is God, and none stands by Him.

For My thoughts are not your thoughts, neither are your ways My ways, saith the Lord. For as the heavens are higher than the earth, so are My ways higher than your ways, and My thoughts than your thoughts. For as the rain cometh down, and the snow from heaven, and returneth not thither, but watereth the earth, and maketh it bring forth and bud, that it may give seed to the sower, and bread to the eater: So shall My words be that goeth forth out of My mouth: it shall not return unto Me void, but it shall accomplish that which I please, and it shall prosper in the thing whereto I sent it.

We thank and praise you Lord. You are God and we are your people. You have created us in your image and made us a little lower than you, that we might create as you have. We thank you that after you called Adam, man, you had him to call woman, Eve, and every creature of the earth. Your spirit dwells within us that we may be like you. That we might have dominion over the earth. That we be god on earth. That we be joint-heirs with Christ Jesus, through the blood of Christ. Children of God. The favored of God. The righteousness of God. All things come of thee, Oh Lord.

We thank you that we have the free gift of salvation. We have been redeemed from destruction. Brought with a price. The price of your blood on Calvary. We thank you, that we have a blood bought right to be free.

Those that the Son sets free, are free indeed. That we are out of debt, with our needs met and plenty more to put in store. We'll never be broke another day in our lives! We are blessed to be a blessing to all nations of the earth.

We thank you that you are Jehovah Jireh, our provision as we go through life. We thank you that you are Jehovah Nissi, our banner in times of need. We thank you that you are Jehovah Gmolah, our recompense of reward. We thank you that you are Jehovah Shammah, you are always there for us in good and bad times. We thank you that you are Jehovah Shalom. Our peace, the one who gives wholeness, nothing missing and nothing broken. We thank you that you are Jehovah Rophe, our healer. We thank you that you are Jehovah M'Kaddesh, the one who sanctifies. It is your word that cleanses us and shows us the way, truth and life. We thank you that you are Jehovah Tsidkenu, you are our righteousness.

You are more than enough to meet every need and want. You are the Almighty God, El Shaddai. We thank you for supernatural increase. We thank you for the favor of God that produces supernatural increase in the seeds we plant into good ground. We thank you for the favor of God that produced increase assets especially in the realm of real estate. We thank you for the favor that produces battles won, that we don't have to fight. We thank you for increase in our family. That the love and respect will grow from heart to heart and breast to breast. We thank you for increase on our job. All that we do is as unto you, Lord. We thank you for increase in our business. That you will give us the Rhema word we need to press forward into your will for our lives. We thank you for the increase and favor when we seem unlikely to receive. We thank you for the increase in our study time. We thank you for the favor of God that produced legislation and rules to be changed in our favor.

We thank you that all your promises are ye and Amen. We thank you that you promised that none of your words will return unto you void, but will accomplish all that you sent them forth to do. That no weapon formed against us shall prosper. That every tongue that rise up against us shall be condemned. Greater is He that is in us than he than is in the world. I can do all things through Christ that strengthens me. By Jesus' stripes I am healed. I will be a lender and not a borrower all the days of my life. God is no respecter of persons. That I will meditate on thy word day and night that I may make my way prosperous and have good success. That wealth and riches are in my houses Now! He will not suffer thy foot to be moved: He that keepeth Isreal shall neither slumber nor sleep. The Lord is thy keeper: the Lord is thy shade upon thy right hand. Ye, though I walk through the valley of the shadow of death, I will fear no evil: for thou art with me; thy rod and thy staff they comfort me. Thou prepare a table before me in the presence of my enemies. Thou anoints my head with oil, my cup runeth over. Surely, Goodness and Mercy shall follow me all the days of my life and I will dwell in the house of the Lord forever.

Blessed is the man that walks not in the counsel of the ungodly, nor stands in the way of sinners, nor sits in the seat of the scornful. But his delight is in the law of the Lord; and in his law doth he meditate day and night. And he shall be like a tree planted by the rivers of water, that brings forth his fruit in his season; his leaf also shall not wither; and whatsoever he does shall prosper. The hand of the diligent shall bear rule: but the slothful shall be under tribute. He becomes poor that deals with a slack hand: but the hand of the diligent maketh rich. The slothful man roasts not that which he took in hunting: But the substance of the diligent man is precious. The soul of the sluggard desires, and hath nothing: but the soul of the diligent shall be made fat. The thoughts of the diligent tend only to plenteousness; but of every one that is hasty(rash or impatient) only to want. See thou a man diligent in his business? He shall stand before kings; he shall not stand before mean men.

We thank you that we can choose life, blessings and prosperity. And we thank you for the word that has showed us your will in our lives. We thank you for your Spirit that He comforts us. He leads and guides us through your word. He reveals mysteries to us. He brings back to our remembrance Rhema word to helps us and gives us the power to get wealth. He is the power of healing. He is the power to deliver. He is our teacher for revelation. We thank you that He prays for us in secrets that you can understand, that is for our benefit.

We thank you that Money! Cometh, to me, Now! Hallelujah. Money! Cometh, to me, Now! Hallelujah! Millions!!! Cometh, to me, Now! Hallelujah! Hallelujah! Hallelujah! Praise be unto our God, for He is worthy to be praised. From the rising of the sun to the going down of the same. He is worthy, Jesus is worthy to be praised. For His Word, His Truth, His Mercy, His Power and His Love endures forever.

He that dwells in the secret place of the most High shall abide under the shadow of the Almighty. I will say of the Lord, He is my refuge and my fortress: my God; in Him will I trust. Surely He shall deliver thee from the snare of the fowler, and from the noisome pestilence. He shall cover thee with His feathers, and under His wings shalt thou trust: His truth shall be thy shield and buckler. Thou shalt not be afraid for the terror by night; nor for the arrow that flieth by day; Nor for the pestilence that walketh in darkness; nor for the destruction that wasteth at noonday. A thousand shall fall at thy side. And ten thousand at thy right hand; but it shall not come night thee. Only with thine eyes shalt thou behold and see the reward of the wicked. Because thou hast made the Lord, which is my refuge, even the most High, thy habitation; There shall no evil befall thee, neither shall any plague come nigh thy dwelling. For He shall give His angels charge over thee, to keep thee in all thy ways. They shall bear thee up in their hands, lest thou dash thy foot against a stone. Thou shalt tread upon the lion and adder: the young lion and the dragon shalt thou trample under feet. Because he hath set his love upon Me, therefore will I deliver him: I will set him on high, because He hath known My Name. He shall call upon Me and I will answer him: I will be with him in trouble; I will deliver him, and honor him. With long life will I satisfy him, and shew him My salvation. To God be the Glory, Amen.

Read once a day, to encourage yourself in the word of God, and renew your strength Calling those things that be not, as though they are.

The Root of Evil

So many sins stems from the love of or the lack of money.

Example: Disobedient children

1. Parents to busy working for money to spend time with them and show them that they love them, so the children rebel.
2. Parents that lack money teach their children; to lie, steal, covet, fornicate, kill, and commit adultery.

    Lie to creditors, "Tell them I'm not home"

    Steal from God, "I'm not giving 10%, of my money, to that preacher"

Covet others peoples things since you can not afford your own

Fornicate by Keeping a man or woman that you won't marry to help you with your financial needs

Kill by Dogging out people on your job, to get the promotion over them

Commit adultery by Being to busy to satisfy your spouse's needs and cause them to have a wondering eye

Or your out of the house so much, that you think you need someone on the side while you are in the street, so called working

Proverb 22:6 says Train up a child in the way he should go and when he is old he won't depart from it. You church people, that have these way-ward children had some form or some degree of the things I just mentioned going on in your house. Now, if your taking your child to church, they know what your suppose to be doing, but if they never see you doing it, they will decide that church either does not work so, why should they go? Or if they go, they will go after a night of sinning or before a day of unrighteousness.

Romans 12:1-2 I beseech you therefore, (Brothers and Sisters), by the mercies of God, that you present your bodies a living sacrifice, holy, acceptable unto God,

which is your reasonable service, And be not conformed to this world: but be ye transformed by the renewing of your mind, that ye may prove what is that good, and acceptable, and perfect will of God.

To be able to present your bodies a living sacrifice you'll need to die to your flesh, give up your carnal living and seek God's purpose for your life. Accept that God made you righteous. God made you righteous. God made you Righteous. **You did not have to work for that righteousness.** Jesus, has already done the work, you just have to step up and receive your new position. You don't have to pray to get righteous. Righteous people pray. You don't have to fast to get righteous. Righteous people fast. You don't have praise God to be righteous. Righteous people praise God.

Please, don't confess that false humility, that you are just a filthy rag, or you are a sinner save by grace, or unworthy. When you accepted Jesus Christ as your Lord and Savior, and confessed your sins, He cleaned you up. Before you accepted Jesus you **were** a sinner, after you accepted Him you were saved from sin so, you are no longer a sinner you **are** the **Righteousness of God.**

Salvation is of God, but you have to choose to accept your new status and die to your flesh, obey God's word and He will sanctify you. To be Holy is to agree with God and obey the word you hear. When God made you the righteousness of God, He gave you the authority to come boldly to the Throne of Grace. So, why say unworthy. If you can come in God's presence, what could you possibly be unworthy to do? Being in God's presence is everything! In the presence of God is healing, peace, joy, deliverance and your inheritance.

God wants you to have money, He just does not want you to have a wrong relationship with money. He has so, many promises in His word, that if you line up with Him, you will receive all of what Jesus died to get to you. Whether or not, you feel you need money is irrelevant. God has a demand on the money to do what He called us to do with it. ***1Timothy 6:17-19 Charge them that are***

rich in this world, that they be not high minded, nor trust in uncertain riches, but in the living God, who giveth us richly all things to enjoy; That they do good, that they be rich in good works, ready to distribute, willing to communicate; Lay up in store for them selves a good foundation against the time to come, that they may lay hold on eternal life.

Can you see in this scripture that God is saying do good, then He goes on to give examples of doing good. Rich in good works, to reiterate the good works, ready to distribute, (sowing into good ground,) and willing to communicate. Philippians 4:15-19. Explains how the church of Philippi communicated with Paul with their money.

Now, if you have not been faithful in your giving to the house of God or the man of God to forward the ministry, don't expect ***God to supply all your needs according to His riches in glory by Christ Jesus.*** Also, just because you claim poverty don't even think your exempt. ***Hebrews 13:15-16 Offer to God the sacrificial fruit of our lips and fruit of our hands: for with such sacrifices God is well pleased.***

Answer me this one question: Do you think God is unfair? Have you sometimes wondered why God would want you to take a vow of poverty then turn around and ask you for money, knowing you don't have any? If God wanted you to be poverty stricken, He would not think of asking you for anything. I submit to you, that the thought of living on crumbs and having just enough to supply your own needs, **is of the devil.** God calls His people to give, of your time, your praise, your prayers, your faithfulness, your ministry, your witness and resoundingly your money, that it may abound to your account.

How many know that Satan attends church regularly. Just like God comes on the praises of his people. Satan came in with his. God knows that we are in this world, but not of the world, but while we are here, we need money to live. With no money you live on the streets. Or you make yourself a slave to creditors or the government. Taking only what they say you can have, never meeting all of your needs. So, where is the abundant life that Jesus died for us to have?

God has never ask us to do anything without compensation. He is Jehovah Gmolah. ***Remember Galatians 6:7*** If you say, that God asked you to work or to give expecting nothing, that would suggest that God is taking advantage of you. A quick example; How would you feel if after a weeks worth of work, your employer says, thanks, great job, see you next week, with just a hand shake and no check? You would put down your religion so quick. Next question: How long will you keep that job? If God never compensated you, you would think of

God as a tyrant, one who takes and never gives, but if it's more blessed to give that to receive, are we more blessed than God? God forbid.

So, in the same token if you don't expect anything from God, after while you'll convince yourself its not worth the trouble to give; so you won't witness to anyone, you won't study to show yourself approved unto God, you won't pray one for another, you won't fellowship with any of the ministries in the church and you definitely won't give any money. In fact you will develop a "What have you done for me lately," attitude towards giving. But it's not really towards giving, it's towards God, since He said to give.

Clueless and trying to sound holy or spiritual, people block their own blessings of God by not giving, saying crazy things **against** their harvest, and the worst of all, not knowing how to **receive a blessing.** Don't you know, when you refuse a gift or a blessing you are stopping the other person from giving. In a false attempt to be, '**more blessed**.' Wake up! God is not impressed with your self-righteousness.

Wrong thinking and wrong relationship with money will cause you to drive a wedge between you and God. The love of money is the root of all evil. Until you get this money situation together your going to continue to have problems, your going to continue to disobey God and you're going to live a miserable life. ***John 10:10 says, It's the thief that comes not, but to steal, and to kill, and to destroy: I am come that they might have life, and that they might have it more abundantly.*** If Jesus died that you have more than enough, why are you trying to settle for just enough, that quickly becomes not enough, as soon as; the car breaks down, rent goes up, a tooth breaks, school pictures are due, children graduate, family members get married, you get an invitation to a birthday party, run out of gas, you get stressed at your job and need a vacation or someone goes on to be with the Lord.

What you forget is, these things are going to happen whether you are prepared for them or not. So, why not take God up on His offer in ***Malachi 3:10 Bring the whole tithe into the store house, that there may be food in My house. Test Me in this, says the Lord Almighty and see if I will not open you the windows of heaven, an pour you out a blessing, that you will not have room enough to receive it.*** Then, communicate with your church, sow into the lives of those in need, sow your tithe and offering, ***give that it shall be given unto you, good measure, pressed down, and shaken together, and running over, shall men give unto your bosom. Luke 6:38.*** God promises when you honor Him he will not only give back to you multiplied, but He will also, ***(v11) rebuke the devourer.*** So, that your money won't be wasted or taken away from you.

God has plans for that money. If the church is called to feed the hungry, clothe the naked, support the homeless, seek the salvation of our kindred and go into all the world spreading the gospel, $5 won't do it. A dollar here, a dollar there won't do it. God needs some multimillionaires to obey and give according as they have so, that the work can get done. If you were out of debt, your needs were met and you had plenty more to put in store, what would your attitude about giving be? Right now, your upset because you barley have enough to meet your needs so, you get mad when someone asks you for something. That being the case, **how will you ever be a cheerful giver?** To be broke is sin.

Stop hating money coming to you, so you can get free and do what Jesus' life example shows us to do. And don't go thinking that, Jesus was poor crap. To be poor means you are **without something**. Jesus had the words to eternal life, what could he possibly be missing? On the material side, He had a house in Capernaum,(the one that the men ripped the roof off of to get into, to see Jesus), Money enough and resources enough to supply the needs of 13 men for 3 ½ years. (the money bag that Judas was suppose to be treasurer of, but was stealing from all along, and no one knew but Jesus, since they never ran out)

How do you think that Jesus could keep the peace that He has? There was nothing missing and nothing broken. God said, in ***Matthew 6:33 seek ye first the kingdom of God and His Righteousness; and all these things will be added unto you.*** All these things were all the things we need to live on the earth; money, clothes, food and shelter. God wants us to have these things. More importantly, He wants us to put them in their proper place. Take note, Solomon asked for wisdom(things of God) and God gave him everything else as a bonus. Romans 8:32 says, God already gave His best gift which is

Christ Jesus, why do you think God would be so tight with the money. **God is not broke.** The earth is the Lords and the fulness there of. Change your thinking, renew your mind. ***Let this mind be in you which is also, in Christ Jesus.***

God wants you to give so that the gospel can go throughout the world. It's not **just** so that your pastor can drive a new car. If he is faithful to God and your church is prosperous there is no reason, that your pastor should have to drive 'Bessie' around. You, looking good and your pastor looking good is a testimony to the goodness of God. **You and your pastor looking broke, busted and disgusted is a testimony to unbelievers not**

to get involved with that church stuff, you'll start to look like them. Please, before you look all good and your pastor looks all good, **make sure you have taken care of God's house first,** then God can open up a window of heaven and pore you all out a blessing that you have not room to receive.

Let me ask you a question: How long do you want to stay here, on this earth, with the evil that's all about us? How long do you want to be attacked by the prince of this world? We have the power to hit the devil where he lives, cut him off at the root of sin, by changing our minds about money. Let the righteousness of God take control over the unrighteous mammon. Let our money be on a mission, to do the work of God, on the earth so, that all the nations of the earth can be blessed. Then Jesus can come and get us out of here!!!

Hallelujah! Hallelujah! Hallelujah! To His Name.

God…Can you hear me?

I Guess today with all the lawlessness and dispar, the overwhelming question on church goers mind **is, God… Can you hear me?** The answer is yes. Now consider the answer, that God is putting back to you. ***If my people, who are called by my name, would humble themselves, and pray, and seek my face, and turn from their wicked ways; then will I hear from heaven, and will forgive their sin, and will heal their land.***

2 Chronicles 7:14 And that's a promise. You know all of God's promises are ye and amen. So, the problem is not with God. It's with us. Why do we continually try to make God give us the life we want, instead of accepting the life that Jesus died for us to have, that includes all of the things we say we want and the things we won't mention in public that we desire. ***John 10:10 says, It's the thief that comes not, but to steal, and to kill, and to destroy: I am come that they might have life, and that they might have it more abundantly.***

Have you ever noticed that when it comes to us, the Bible always says things like **might** and **If**, but all of Gods promises are definite. So, why are we not living the abundant life when God's words are definite and true? Well, Jesus said, ***Learn of Me for my yoke is easy, and my burden is light,*** but church goers believe the world's word over God's word. So, they chose the burden and yoke of the world's system. Now listen to the insanity, they pray to God for help while they reject His Word and Way and think that prayer doesn't work. **Hello!** God has a system in place that if we line up with it we will **receive** what God says we can have. You cannot mix the two. God has no fellowship with the devil. You cannot think and act like the world and receive the full benefits of Gods system.

Be not deceive. God is not mocked. Whatsoever, you sow, that you will also reap. (Galatians 6:7) You cannot plant apple seeds and get a peach tree. In the same token you cannot sow unto the flesh and reap life.

Sowing to the flesh will only bring corruption and death. Just like sowing to the spirit will produce blessings and life. It's a choice. God does not make you do anything, but He has set before you the options of Life and Death. ***Deuteronomy 30:19 states, I call heaven and earth to record this day against you, that I have set before you life and death, blessings and curses, therefore, chose life that you and your children may live.*** He set before us a no brain-er multiple choice question, and then gave us the answer. And people still look to God and blame Him for all the trouble in their lives.

Compliance to the word of God, will cause God to move on your behalf to bring to pass His word in your life. He is not obligated to bring your word to pass. Get that into your spirit. I think I'll say it again, **God is not obligated to bring your word to pass.** He only promised that His word will not return unto Him void, but it will accomplish all that He sent it to do.

Some people believe, that some people are destined to be blessed, above others and some are destined to be poor. That is a lie from the pit of hell and I will prove it with 5 scriptures:

1. *Acts 10:34 Peter said of a truth, I perceive that God is not a respecter of persons*
2. *Psalms 35:27 Let the Lord be magnified that takes pleasure in the prosperity of His servants*
3. *Deuteronomy 8:18 Remember the Lord thy God: it is He that gives you the power to get wealth*
4. *3 John 2 Beloved I wish above all things that you prosper and be in health*
5. *John 10:10 (Jesus) came that we might have life, and have it more abundantly*

Now, we have to receive those words. If you don't accept the word of God, it will not work in your life. The word says, ***a double minded man is unstable in all his ways, and he should not expect anything from God. (James 1:7-8)*** Christian on Sunday and worker of iniquity on Monday is double mindedness. I love you today, but scandalize your name tomorrow is double mindedness. Pastor thank you for your prayers on Tuesday, guess what Suzy, Pastor and Sis. Jones left my house together last Tuesday, double mindedness. ***Bitter and sweet waters should not come from the same spring.(James 3:10-11)***

Check your self, before you wreck your self. A phrase that the children use, ironically enough, its biblical. God wants us to accept the new creature that He is making us into through His word. He wants us to walk in the Favor of God, and live that abundant life, that Jesus gave His life, for us to have. When you start to obey the word of God, you will find that first, God will instruct you on the changes that need to be made. As the changes begin to occur, then you can call on God for things or answers, and you will find them there immediately. You will not have to wait two and three years for God to answer. Fellowship with God is like that. You can ask God for something that morning and before lunch it is there, **when you are obedient to His word.** ***Jesus said, If ye abide in me, and my words abide in you, ye shall ask what ye will, and it shall be done unto you. John 15:7*** Remember, that will only come after the purging. The purging is to put you on the same page with Jesus. To receive the mantle from Elijah, Elisha had to see things eye to eye with Elijah. For us today to receive anything from the Father, we must to see things eye to eye with Jesus(The Word of God). I won't lie to you the purging will hurt your flesh. If you are willing and obedient, and allow the destruction of your flesh and all of it's worldly desires you to be brought to naught, you will be able to experience the, it shall be done unto you, part of God.

See, you thought that, you could do what you wanted to do, serve Satan and beg God for things. **No, its not like that.** You get rewarded from your God. If you are acting like Satan, then ask him for the desires of your heart. Since, he is the god you are serving. Its like dealing with your parents, If you clean your room, do your homework and get good grades, you can ask your parents for anything, at their pocket level. But, if you are a screw-up in school, get rotten grades and stay in the detention hall, for one reason or the other. You are not going to get your parents to go and get you the desires of your heart. Ask your friends that you were influenced by to get it. The only difference between God and your parents is, the earth is the Lords and the fullness thereof, so, God does not have a limit on what you can ask Him for, if your lined up with His word.

Isn't God Awesome. He is so Wonderful. He is Excellent in all that He does. He won't short change you. You heard that the word says, that ***God watches over His word to perform it.*** He is ready, willing and able to give you all that you want. He will even go exceeding and abundantly beyond, what you can ask or think. So, repent to God, get lined up with His word and then call on His Rich and Holy name, and see if He can hear you.

Love…The action word of God

For God so loved the world, that He gave His only begotten Son, that whosoever believeth in Him should not perish, but have everlasting life. For God sent not His Son into the world to condemn the world: but that the world through Him might be saved. John 3:16-17Niv This is my commandment, that ye love one another, as I have loved you. Greater love hath no man than this, that a man lay down his life for his friends. Ye are my friends, if ye do whatsoever I command you. Henceforth I call you not servants; for the servant knows not what his lord does: but I have called you friends; for all things that I

have heard of my Father I have made known unto you. Ye have not chosen me, but I have chosen you, and ordained you, that you should go and bring forth fruit, and that your fruit should remain: that whatsoever ye shall ask of the Father in my name, He may give it you. John15:12-16 God has no problem showing us His love. His love always leaves us in a better position than we started. Throughout His word, He shows us how to say I love you to others, with our actions.

1 Corinthians 13:4-8aNiv Love is patient, love is kind. It does not envy, it does not boast, it is not proud. It is not rude, it is not self-seeking, it is not easily angered, it keeps no record of wrongs. Love does not delight in

evil, but rejoices with the truth. It always protects, always trusts, always hopes, always perseveres. Love never fails.

Matthew 5:43-48Niv You have heard that it was said, 'Love your neighbor and hate your enemy.' But I tell you: Love your enemies and pray for those who persecute you, that you may be sons of your Father in heaven, He causes His sun to rise on the evil and the good, and sends rain on the righteous and the unrighteous. If you love those who love you, what reward will you get? Are not even the tax collectors doing that? And if you greet only your brothers, what are you doing more than others? Do not even pagans do that? Be perfect, therefore, as your heavenly Father is perfect.

Proverbs 10: 11-12 The mouth of the righteous is a fountain of life, but violence overwhelms the mouth of the wicked, Hatred stirs up strife: but love covers all sins.

Proverbs 15:17 Better a meal of vegetables where there is love, than a fattened calf with hatred.

Ephesians 4:17- 5:2Niv So I tell you this, and insist on it in the Lord, that you must no longer live as the Gentiles do, in the futility of their thinking. They are darkened in their understanding and separated from the life of God because of the ignorance that is in them due to the hardening of their hearts. Having lost all sensitivity, they have given themselves over to sensuality so as to indulge in every kind of impurity, with a continual lust for more.

You, however, did not come to know Christ that way. Surely you heard of Him and were taught in Him in accordance with the truth that is in Jesus. You were taught, with regard to your former way of life, to put off your old self, which is being corrupted by its deceitful desires; to be made new in the attitude of your minds; and to put on the new self, created to be like God in true righteousness and holiness.

v25 Therefore, each of you must put off falsehood and speak truthfully to his neighbor, for we are all members of one body. "In your anger do not sin" Do not let the sun go down while you are still angry, and do not give the devil a foothold. He who has been stealing must steal no longer, but must work doing something useful with his own hands, that he may have something to share with those in need.

v29 Do not let any unwholesome talk come out of your mouth, but only what is helpful for building others up according to their needs, that it may benefit those who listen. And do not grieve the Holy Spirit of God, with whom you were sealed for the day of redemption. Get rid of all bitterness, rage and anger, brawling and slander, along with every form of malice. Be kind and compassionate to one another, forgiving each other, just as in Christ God forgave you.

5v1 Be imitators of God. therefore, as dearly loved children and live a life of love, just as Christ loved us and gave himself up for us as a fragrant offering and sacrifice to God.

1 John 4:7-21Niv Dear friends, let us love one another, for love comes from God. Everyone who loves has been born of God and knows God. Whoever does not love does not know God, because God is love. This is how God showed His love among us: He sent His one and only Son in the world that we might live through Him. This is love: not that we loved God, but that He loved us and sent His Son as an atoning sacrifice for our sins. Dear friends, since God so loved us, we also ought to love one another. No one has ever seen God; but if we love one another, God lives in us and His love is made complete in us.

We know that we live in Him and He in us, because He has given us of His Spirit. And we have seen and testify that the Father has sent His Son to be the Savior of the world. If anyone acknowledges that Jesus is the Son of God, God lives in him and he is in God. And so we know and rely on the love God has for us.

God is love. Whoever lives in love lives in God, and God in him. In this way love is made complete among us so that we will have confidence on the day of judgment, because in this world we are like Him. <u>There is no fear in</u>

love. But perfect love drives out fear, because fear has torment. The one who fears is not made perfect in love.

We love because He first loved us. If anyone says, "I love God," yet hates his brother, he is a liar. For anyone who does not love his brother, whom he has seen, cannot love God, whom he has not seen. And He has given us this command: Whoever loves God must also love his brother.

I Peter 4Niv Therefore, since Christ suffered in His body, arm yourselves also with the same attitude, because He who has suffered in His body is done with sin. As a result, He does not live the rest of His earthly life for evil human desires, but rather for the will of God.

For you have spent enough time in the past doing what pagans choose to do - living in debauchery, lust, drunkenness, orgies, carousing and detestable idolatry. They think it strange that you do not plunge with them into the same flood of dissipation, and they heap abuse on you. But they will have to give account to Him who is ready to judge the living and the dead. For this is the reason the gospel was preached even to those who are now dead, so that they might be judged according to men regard to the body, but live according to God in regard to the spirit. The end of all things is near. <u>Therefore be clear minded and self-controlled so that you can pray.</u> Above all, love each other deeply, *because love covers over a multitude of sins. Offer hospitality to one another without grumbling. Each one should use whatever gift he has received to serve others, faithfully administering God's grace in its various forms. If anyone speaks, he should do it as one speaking the very words of God. If any one serves, he should do it with the strength God provides, so that in all things God may be praised through Jesus Christ. To Him be the glory and the power for ever and ever. Amen.*

Notice our love shows through greater in the kind and caring way we respond to peoples needs. Even people who are hard to get along with, need someone to just accept them for who they are and just love them, by not making a big deal of their shortcomings. God said, what benefit is it to you to just treat those good who treat you good. Even the sinners do that? What reward do you expect only doing just enough? **God calls us to be outstanding.** As He puts it, a peculiar people, separated; called out; sanctified; Holy; the Righteousness of God. You won't get there doing just enough. You should want to do like God does, exceeding and abundantly beyond all you can ask or think.

When you let the love flow from heart to heart and breast to breast you can seriously impact some peoples lives. God blesses us so, that we can be a blessing to all nations of the earth. You can smile all day long, pray all day long, sit and say you understand all day long, but when you pull out a check book and help a person that lost their job keep their home, you'll make them Holla! They will love God for giving you the thought to bless them, they will love you for your obedience, they will love their family more since they don't have to look at their sad faces anymore and you will love how you feel that you'll want to go and show some more love and bless some more people. Make sure, its by God's leadership, and all will turn out great.

How to internalize the Word of God

There are some things you'll need to know, understand and receive about God and His word to be able to internalize them. If you want to have a closer and more intimate relationship with God you will need to learn about Him and get to know His thoughts about things. Learn how he fells about the things we say, do and how our actions effect our relationship with Him. You may want to get a closer look at His character. Well how can I do that? ***Learn of Him, for His yoke is easy and His burden is light.*** ***You will also need to study to show yourself*** *approved of God, a workman that needs not to be ashamed rightly dividing the words of truth. (ref. Matthew 11:30 & 2 Timothy 2:15)*

First, God is a spirit. *John 4:24 God is a spirit and they that worship Him, must worship Him in spirit and truth.* What is worship? In Genesis 22:5 Abraham described worship as doing what God told him to do. Holiness is described the exact same way. Being in agreement with God in speech and actions. You cannot forget the action part. *Be ye doers of the word and not hearers only, deceiving yourself. James 1:22* We are spiritual beings, we have a soul and a flesh case to cover. To be led by the spirit is to die to the fleshly wants and needs.

You will need to strive to be totally obedient to the Spirit of God within you. Therefore, to put it all together as we study the word and see our short comings, we will have to choose the way of the Spirit of God, to be delivered from those old ways. To worship God is to let them go and cleave to the new way of life that He is showing us, that we can have by obedience to Him.

Secondly, God is the Word. *John 1:1-5 In the beginning was the Word, and the Word was with God, and the Word was God. The same was in the beginning with God. All things were made by him; and without him was not anything made that was made. In him was life; and the life was the light of men. And the light shines in darkness; and the darkness comprehended it not. v10-14 He was in the world, and the world was made by him, and the world knew Him not. He came unto his own, and His own received Him not. But as many as received Him, to them gave He power to become the sons of God, even to them that believe on His name: Which were born, not of blood, nor of the will of the flesh, nor of the will of man, but of God. And the Word was made flesh, and dwelt among us, (and we beheld His glory, the glory as of the only begotten of the Father,) full of grace and truth.*

Read of Him for yourself. I don't believe you can have a close, personal and intimate relationship with someone thru a third party. The preacher can't show you the love of God through his words. He does not have the vocabulary to explain the dept, height and width of God and His love. The preacher cannot put into words the compassion, healing or mercy of God. For him to try, would be like, trying to describe to you, while you stand hot, on a desert, what a tall glass of icy water would taste and feel like, while your watching him drink it. You would not want him to explain how it tastes, you would want to experience it for yourself.

If you are lazy and only want to hear the preacher talk about heaven, you are missing out on the heaven here on earth that Jesus died to get to you. ***The thief cometh***

not, but to steal, and to kill, and to destroy: I am come that they might have life, and that they might have it more abundantly. John 10:10 Notice the **might**, it is not automatic. You will need to believe the word is true, receive it and get with God to live it. Heaven represents being in the presence of God. There is no better place on earth to be. Remember, when you worship God continually you bask in the presence of God. I can't explain it and do it justice, so, I won't try. All I have to say is, please take God up on His offer to walk in His presences.

Third, **God is power.** He is the ability to do every thing that has to be done. The power to create the world, the power to cause and old woman to conceive and bear a child of promise. He is the power to change plain cows to speckled, spotted and stripped ones. He is the power to deliver Joseph from the pit to the palace and build the wealth foundation, that will supply the Israelites the reward for 400 years of slavery. He is the power to deliver them from Egypt with nothing missing and nothing broken, through the red sea on dry land, sustain them while in the wilderness for 40 years, give them manna from the sky, water from a rock and open up the earth to get rid of the rubbish. He parted the Jordan, tore down the walls of Jericho, defeated the enemies, stopped the earth to complete the battle and is able to make you prosperous and have good success. He raised up Samuel, anointed David and protected Him from Saul, prospered Solomon and built the temple, took Elijah, healed Naaman, and added fifteen years to Hezekiah's life. Defeated the enemy with the praise of His people, restored Job double what he lost, makes us to rest in the shadow of the Almighty and makes His word accomplish all that He sent it forth to do. He put His words in the mouth of Jeremiah, He made dry bones live before Ezekiel, He protected Daniel and the three Hebrew boys from the kings of Babylon, He taught Hosea about love, He gave Joel vision and to Amos He gave prophesy of the Lord. He gave to Jonah direction and to Malachi the ability to rebuke the devourer. He protected the seed of promise for 42 generations, gave Him the ability to heal the sick, raise the dead, give sight to the blind, fed 5000 with a small boys lunch, made the transference of righteousness with sinful man, tore down the temple and raised Him up in three days. Someone aught to say Glory! Praise be unto our God for He is the Almighty God, El Shaddai.

Now that you know who God is and what He is capable of doing, build on those words daily with your own testimony of God's deliverance in your life and the lives of others. Put it in your ears, your eyes and get it into your spirit. Become personally acquainted with God by staying in constant contact with Him. He is everywhere and in every aspect of your life. ***Ask and it shall be given you; seek, and you shall find; knock, and it shall be opened unto you: For every one that asketh receiveth; and he that seeketh findeth; and to him that knocketh it shall be opened. Matthew 7:7-8*** Do a combination of the following list at least once a day:

1. *Put it in your ears. Rom 10:17 So then faith cometh by hearing, and hearing by the word of God.*
2. *Put it in front of your eyes. Deuteronomy 17:19 And it shall be with him, and he shall read*

therein all the days of his life: that he may learn to fear the Lord his God, to keep all the words of this law and these statutes, to do them:

3. *Study to help them sink down into your spirit. 2 Timothy 2:15 Study to show thy self approved of God, a workman that needeth not to be ashamed, rightly dividing the words of truth.*
4. *Recognize the value of the word. Matthew 4:4 But He answered and said, it is written, Man shall not live by bread alone, but by every word that proceedeth out of the mouth of God.*

5. Memorize the word. Ps 119:11 Thy word have I hid in mine heart, that I might not sin against thee.

6. Meditate on the word. Joshua 1:8 This book of the law shall not depart out of thy mouth; but thou shalt meditate therein day and night, that thou mayest observe to do according to all that is written there in: for then thou shalt make thy way prosperous, and then thou shalt have good success.

7. Live the word. James 1:22 But be ye doers of the word, and not hearers only, deceiving your own selves.

Experience God in some shape or form every day. Seek Him while He can be found. Look for Him in every aspect of your life. Give Him the credit for every thing He does in your life. Listen when He speaks to you thru His word. Speak His word that He may be able to bring it to pass in your life. And do it continually. Remember, the key is **stability**. Don't treat Him like you treat mom, give me, give me, give me. Be quick to give Him all the praise, honor, and adoration that He is due. And watch Him blow your mind and leave you in awe of Him.

I am in covenant with God

Get a hold on to that. I am in covenant with The Almighty God, who is able to do exceedingly and abundantly above all I can ask or think. We must seek to find out what the covenant is, why it was so important and what all of it means for us today. God had it all together before time was. He is truly awesome and as we get into this, you will get in agreement with me about how phenomenal God is.

First, what is a covenant? A covenant is an agreement between two or more parties. An agreement that joins them in order to cancel out the weakness of both making one strong unit. A ceremony takes place to signify the union and exchange of the names and coats. That exchange lets the world know about the covenant and that caution should be taken when an attempt to attack one or the other is being formulated.

The following is an example:

A farmer family named Smith and a warrior family named Fields, want to join in covenant. The heads meet and discuss their weakness and how the union could erase both of their weaknesses. The farmers are being attacked, their harvest has been stolen by thieves and they are powerless to defend against the mob. The warriors often find themselves weakened due to lack of nourishment. If they join forces the farmers could provide the nourishment for the warrior and the warrior would give protection of their harvest. They agree.

At the ceremony they sacrifice animals to supply the blood. As they walk through the blood they confess their promises to one another. The farmer says you will never be hungry another day in your life. I will give myself as food before I allow you to go hungry. The warrior says you will never be robbed another day in your life. I will fight to the death for your safety. Now the name exchange, they are no longer the Smiths and Fields they are the Smithfields. They exchange coats now to signify to the world that they are in covenant together. In blood covenant nothing can break it but death.

In Genesis 17, God called Abram to join in covenant with Him. *v1-2(Niv) When Abram was ninety-nine years old the lord appeared to Abram, and said to him, "I am the Almighty God; walk before me and be thou perfect. And I will make my covenant between Me and thee, and I will multiply thee exceedingly." v6-7 "And I will make thee exceedingly fruitful, and I will make nations of thee, and kings shall come out of thee. And I will establish my covenant between me and thee and thy seed after thee in their generations for an everlasting covenant, to be a God unto thee, and to thy seed after thee.*

In Genesis 15 they had the ceremonial blood walk. *v8-18 But Abram said, O Sovereign Lord how can I know that I will gain possession of it?" So the Lord said to him, "Bring me a heifer, a goat and a ram, each three years old, along with a dove an a young pigeon," Abram brought all these to him, cut them in two and arranged the halves opposite each other; the birds, however, he did not cut in half. The birds of prey came down on the carcasses, but Abram drove them away. As the sun was setting, Abram fell into a deep sleep, and a thick and dreadful* darkness came over him. The Lord said to him, "Know for certain that your descendants will be strangers in a country not their own, and they will be enslaved and mistreated four hundred years. But I will punish the nation they serve as slaves, an afterward they will come out with great possessions. You, however, will go to your fathers in peace and be buried at a good old age. In the fourth generation your descendants will come back here, for the sin of the Amorites has not yet reached its full measure. Niv. And it came to pass, that, when the sun went down, and it was dark, behold a smoking furnace, and a burning lamp that passed between those pieces. In the same day the Lord made a covenant with Abram, *saying Unto thy seed have I given this land, from the river of Egypt unto the great river, the river Euphrates: KJV*

In Genesis 17 was the exchange of the names. *v5 Neither shall thy name any more be called Abram, but thy name shall be Abraham; for a father of may nations have I made thee. v15 And God said unto Abraham, "As for Sarai thy wife, thou shalt not call her name Sarai, but Sarah shall her name be. And I will bless her, and give thee a son also of her: yea I will bless her, and she shall be a mother of nations; kings of people shall be of her."*

The exchange of the coat came 42 generations later when the seed arrived on the earth. ***Galatians 3:16 Now to Abraham and his seed were the promises made. He saith not, and to seeds, as of many; but as of one, And to thy seed, which is Christ.*** The exchange was the coat of sin and the coat of righteousness.

II Corinthians 5:21 For He hath made Him to be sin for us, who knew no sin; that we might be made the righteousness of God in Him.

All of this had to be done since, Adam gave up every thing to Satan, all the way up to the thrown of God, but not including it. His sin brought death to the world. (The wages of sin is death.) The problem was his death was not able cover what he did. So, God had to step in and give the sacrificial offering to atone for all. (But the gift of God is eternal life through Christ Jesus our Lord. Romans 6:23) The keys of hell and death was with Satan and no righteous man could go where he is so, God used His covenant with sinful man to supply His need to get to hell. ***Then on the third day Jesus arose from the dead, with the keys of hell and death and with all power in His hands.*** Someone aught to say Hallelujah!!!

Now how do we take part; ***Galatians 3:18-29 For if the inheritance be of the law, it is no more of promise: but God gave it to Abraham by promise. Wherefore then serveth the law? It was added because of*** *transgressions, till the seed should come to whom the promise was made; and it was ordained by angels in the hand of the mediator. Now a mediator is not a mediator of one, but God is one. Is the law then against the promises of God? God forbid: for if there had been a law given which could have given life, verily righteousness should have been by the law. But the scripture hath concluded all under sin, that the promise by faith of Jesus Christ might be given to them that believe. But before faith came, we were kept under the law, shut up unto the faith which should afterwards be revealed. Wherefore the law was our schoolmaster to bring us unto Christ, that we might be justified by faith. But after that faith is come, we are no longer under a schoolmaster. For ye are all the children of God by faith in Christ Jesus. For as many of you as have been baptized into Christ have put on Christ. There is neither Jew nor Greek, there is neither bond nor free, there is neither male nor female: for ye are all one in Christ Jesus. And if ye be Christ's, then are ye Abraham's seed, and heirs according to the promise. KJV*

Hallelujah! Hallelujah! Hallelujah! Hallelujah! Hallelujah! God is truly Awesome. It's said, that if Satan really knew what he was doing, he would have never have crucified the Lord. To bad for him, wonderful opportunity for us, to live that abundant life that Jesus died for us to have.

John 10:10 says, It's the thief that comes not, but to steal, and to kill, and to destroy: I am come that they might have life, and that they might have it more abundantly.

When you accept Jesus as your Lord and Savior, you are in a whole new world. The rules of the game change. Your under the ark of safety. You cannot be held back by prejudice, sex, age, birth deformities or any trick, burden or yoke of the devil. Remember, God said, submit yourself to Him, resist the devil and he will flee. If you remember to praise God continually for what He has done and be obedient to His words, you can have whatsoever you ask for. Just don't ever forget that God blesses you to be a blessing to others.

All of God's promises are ye and Amen to those who are called by His name. Search the scriptures to build your relationship with the one who is able to supply all your needs according to His riches in glory. Obedience is key. He required it of Abraham and He requires it of you. ***John 15:7 If ye abide in me and my words abide in you, ye shall ask what ye will, and it shall be done unto you.***

Thy Will Be Done

Why can't we all just get along? Satan has devised a way to separate the body of Christ. How can that be? ***But every man is tempted, when he is drawn away of his own lusts, and enticed. Then when lust hath conceived, it brings forth sin: and sin, when it is finished, brings forth death.(James 1:14-15)*** For too long Christians have been fighting against one another about doctrine and tradition. Never once consulting with God and His thoughts on the matter. When is God going to be number one in the lives of the people who are called by His name?

There are so many different religions and sects and cults in this world, that the stench of them must be making God sick. Come on people, how is Jesus suppose to come back and find His church without spot or wrinkle, when all of this religion is in the way of the pure Gospel that Jesus brought and preached. Jesus did not have a religious bone in His body, so why are you so hung up on these traditions, ceremonies and who is better than who. To take the religious stance is to take the stance of the Pharisees and Sadducee. We all know, throughout Jesus' ministry they chose the 'devils advocate' posture and accused the brethren on every side. They even went so far as to crucify Jesus and lie about his deliverance from the grave. Do you really want to stand with those guys on Judgment Day? God has no fellowship with the devil so; choose you this day whom you will serve, God or Satan.

Now I beseech you, brethren, by the name of our Lord Jesus Christ, that ye all speak the same thing, and that there be no divisions among you; but that ye be perfectly joined together in the same mind and in the same judgment. For it hath been declared unto me of you, my brethren, by them which are of the house of Chloe, that there are contention among you. Now this I say, that every one of you saith, I am of

Paul(Methodist/Baptist); and I of Apollos (Witness/Muslim); and I Cephas (Pentecostal/Adventist) and I of Christ (Catholic/Apostalitic). Is Christ divided? Was Paul crucified for you? Or were you baptized in the name of Paul? I thank God that I baptized none of you, but Crispus and Gaius; Lest any should say that I had baptized in mine own name. And I baptized also the household of Stephanas: besides, I know not whether I baptized any other. For Christ sent me not to baptize, but to preach the gospel: not with wisdom of words, lest the cross of Christ should be made of none effect. For the preaching of the cross is to them that perish foolishness; but unto us which are saved it is the power of God. For it is written, I will destroy the wisdom of the wise, and will bring to nothing the understanding of the prudent. Where is the wise? Where is the scribe? Where is the disputer of this world? Hath not God made foolish the wisdom of this world? For after that in the wisdom of God the world by wisdom knew not God, it pleased God by the foolishness of preaching to save them that believe. For the Jews require a sigh, and the Greeks seek after wisdom: But we preach Christ crucified, unto the Jews a stumbling block, and unto the Greeks foolishness; But unto them which are called, both Jews and Greeks, Christ the power of God, and the wisdom of God. Because the foolishness of God is wiser than men; and the weakness of God is stronger than men. For ye see your calling, brethren, how that not many wise men after the flesh, not many mighty, not many noble, are called: But God hath chosen the foolish things of the world to confound the wise; and God hath chosen the weak things of the world to confound the things which are mighty; And base things of the world, and things which are despised, hath God chosen, yea and things which are not. To bring to nought things that are: That no flesh should glory in His presence. But of him are ye in Christ Jesus, who of God is made unto us wisdom and righteousness, and sanctification, and redemption: That, according as it is written, He that glorieth, let him glory in the Lord.

And I brethren, when I came to you, came not with excellency of speech or of wisdom, declaring unto you the testimony of God. For I determined not to know anything among you, save Jesus Christ, and Him crucified. And I was with you in weakness, and in fear, and in much trembling. And my speech and my preaching was not with enticing words of man's wisdom, but in demonstration of the Spirit and of power: That your faith should not stand in the wisdom of men, but in the power of God. Howbeit we speak wisdom among them that are perfect: yet not the wisdom of this world, nor of the princes of this world, *that come to naught: But we speak the wisdom of God in a mystery, even the hidden wisdom, which God ordained before the world unto our glory: Which none of the princes of this world knew: for had they known it, they would not have crucified the Lord of glory. But as it is written, Eye hath not seen, nor ear heard, neither have entered into the heart of man, the things which God hath prepared for them that love Him. <u>But God hath revealed them unto us by His Spirit:</u> for the Spirit searcheth all things, yea, the deep things of God. For what man knoweth the things of man, save the spirit of man, which is in him? Even so the things of God knoweth no man, but the Spirit of God. Now we have received, not the spirit* *of the world, but the spirit, which is of God; that we might know the things that are freely given to us of God. Which things also we speak, not in the words which man's wisdom teacheth, but which the Holy Ghost teacheth; comparing spiritual things with spiritual. But the natural man receiveth not the things of the Spirit of God: for they are foolishness unto him: neither can he know them, because they are spiritually discerned. But he that is spiritual judgeth all things, yet He Himself is judged of no man. For who hath known the mind of the Lord, that he may instruct Him? But we have the mind of Christ. (1Corinthians 1:10-2:16*

God has a system in place and He sent His Word to the world for His children to learn of it, that they may be able to spread it throughout all nations. When the word goes forth, without dissension and confusion, the body will be joined together. Once we have put aside all backbiting, clamor and malice, without such, the true unadulterated, Word of God, Love of God and Peace of God can flow. Then, unbelievers will see how great we treat one another and want to be apart of the fold. Once all the nations of the earth are blessed by the word, then Jesus can come for a church without a spot or wrinkle. When we get home away from all the death, pain and crying, God will be our God and we will be His people and everything will be as it should be. Glory be unto our God!!! Hallelujah! Hallelujah! Hallelujah!!! Amen.

Bibliography

Scriptures: Mostly Old and New King James Version of the Bible

Scriptures: New International Version of the Bible

Scriptures: The Amplified Version of the Bible

Various Bible Teachings over the years by:

Dr. Creflo Dollar Ministries

World Changers Church International

2500 Burdette Road

College Park, Georgia USA

(888)236-8846

Now That I Am Saved... What Next?
Go to the Next Level

Notes

Notes

Notes

Notes

Notes

Notes

D. Vanessa Smith

Notes

To God be the Glory,

For all the things that He has Done

D. Vanessa Smith

About the Author

So that you know where I'm coming from:

God called me into the fold while I studied His word during the separation of my first marriage. A girlfriend came by to visit me at mommy's place. She saw the noise and confusion going on all around me, and asked me to come and stay with her for a while, just to sort out my feelings and look at my options. I desperately needed peace and quiet to be with *my* thoughts, so, I thought. Therefore, I accepted her offer.

I was a Sunday school teacher, for about eight or nine years, but I did not have a personal relationship with God. I knew Mommy had one, and there were people who were at church that had a relationship with God. I even took the classes to get baptized, although I had not received the understanding of scripture, from the Holy Spirit, at that time. I for the most part, would only read what I had to read, for Sunday school class. Once, I tried to read it straight through like a book, but that did not work. How many of you know, it takes more than just you reading and complaining to have an understanding of scripture?

I did not know, at the time, that the natural man could not understand the ways of God. I was going to church every Sunday, most of the time, after a party or something worst, and I could not understand why, God could not hear my prayers. I did not know that the prayers of the *righteous* availed much. And the only prayer that God wants to hear from a *sinner* is the prayer of *repentance*.

I was blaming my husband for all the wrong that he did during our marriage. I did not consider that he told me before we got married that he was a woman beater. He told me that he had absolutely *no respect* for credit. He also, told me all about people that have hidden agendas for things, but I was not listening. I just wanted to get married, *by any means necessary.* Sound familiar?

I am eternally grateful to God for using her and to Fatima for her obedience to come and offer me a place to stay. I thank and praise God for sending His Spirit to teach me about His Word. I thank and praise Him in advance for all that will be touched by these words and begin a journey toward Jesus. I thank Him for the ones who will see that church attendance is not enough, any more and seek a deeper walk with God. I praise Him for the ones who will have the guts to come out of the shallow waters and go into the deep.

Please address all request for information or permission to:

D. Vanessa Smith
P. O. Box 20313
Newark, New Jersey 07101-6313
E-mail: FirstDNextLevel@aol.com

www.ingramcontent.com/pod-product-compliance
Lightning Source LLC
Chambersburg PA
CBHW030312290526
45785CB00001B/321

* 9 7 8 1 4 0 3 3 8 5 4 2 0 *